GYROSCOPE

A Survival of Sepsis

GARY BLACK

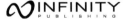
INFINITY
PUBLISHING

ISBN 978-0-7414-6688-4 Paperback
ISBN 978-0-7414-9490-0 eBook
Library of Congress Control Number: 2011930333

Printed in the United States of America

Published March 2012

INFINITY PUBLISHING
1094 New DeHaven Street, Suite 100
West Conshohocken, PA 19428-2713
Toll-free (877) BUY BOOK
Local Phone (610) 941-9999
Fax (610) 941-9959
Info@buybooksontheweb.com
www.buybooksontheweb.com

To my wonderful wife and soul mate Nancy,
for her endless love and support.

CONTENTS

ACKNOWLEDGMENTS

I am deeply indebted to the doctors, nurses, and staff of WakeMed Hospital and WakeMed Rehab. Your kindness, patience, professional performance and dedication helped me to survive and recover from the devastating illness of sepsis. I equally owe a debt of gratitude to Dr. Joseph M. Micchia Jr., who quickly diagnosed my septic condition and rushed me to the Emergency room at the hospital in time for treatment to save my life.

I am also very grateful to my wife, sons, sisters, and other family members and friends for their love, patience, kindness and prayers in my time of need. Their love and support were an integral part of my survival and recovery.

Lastly, with great reverence and appreciation, I thank God for the divine intervention that lifted my body, soul, and spirit back to life from near death.

INTRODUCTION

A wise man should consider that health is the greatest of
human blessings, and learn how by his own thought to
derive benefit from his illness - Hippocrates

Spring blossomed with the promise of summer, and the city
of Raleigh, North Carolina was covered in a powdery blanket of pollen. The months that followed disappeared quickly.
Summer now glared across the soon to be burnt lawns and
untanned bodies with the sweltering Sun Belt heat. Swimming pools opened and vacations began. Yards filled with
kids, dogs, picnics and barbecue smoke.

But I had winter in July. My life was frozen in a cold war
with severe sepsis, and my consciousness of time and the
seasons was transformed into a moment to moment hour to
hour struggle for survival. I did not know that a monster with
a voracious appetite for destruction was waiting to devour
me. It carried with it the capability for raging pain, suffering,
and hopeless despair that would soon thrust me into a lonely
and dark purgatory. My tangible reality was stripped away
and spun off balance like a wobbling gyroscope, while my
spirit, soul, and body fought for survival.

I was overwhelmed. I wouldn't trust anyone except my family. My trembling, fever-ridden body was grossly swollen from

infection, and I gasped to capture each breath. My rational mind had been silenced by the roar of the impending massive Systemic Inflammatory Response Syndrome (SIRS) called sepsis, which may be described as the body's overwhelming auto-destructive response to infection. I became paranoid, delirious, and panic stricken. Beneath my physical symptoms I felt raw fear and anguish. I could sense death's shadowy veil drawing near me, yet I felt the divine presence of love.

This is a true story about surviving sepsis, one of the leading causes of death in the United States. There are approximately 750,000 cases of this mysterious illness each year in the United States, over 200,000 deaths, and it is on the rise. It examines a spectrum of experiences that I endured physically, mentally, and spiritually. My art work illustrates many of the ordeals and episodes that I encountered during my illness and recovery. My research explores the epidemiology of sepsis, and includes some of the latest innovations for treatment, as well as references for further investigation.

I felt compelled to share my experiences to create awareness, increase knowledge, and give helpful insight to the public, patients and their families, and health care professionals who may have already or someday will face this sleeping giant of death and destruction. There is a growing concern for the rise in sepsis cases, their diagnosis and treatment, and the unacceptable mortality rates that accompany it.

I contacted Wake Med Hospital Public Relations at the recommendation of one of my doctors, to get permission to interview hospital staff and use any information such as the hospital name and medical records in my book. I met with Heather Monackey, Senior Public Relations Specialist to review my plan which would include acknowledgements for the fine care I received at Wake Med hospital, as well as excerpts from interviews. She liked my book idea and art work and provided me with an official signed consent form allowing me to proceed. She also patiently helped to set up interviews conducted at the hospital, which included several therapists, a neuropsychologist, and even the executive director of the rehab hospital.

I conducted these interviews with family members, doctors, nurses, therapists and other hospital staff to expand my insight into the events that transpired during my illness. The interviews were hand-written and mailed to me, others were by phone or in person. Some responses were objective and clinical, while others were subjective and emotional. I asked people to describe my physical condition, disposition and behavior, and the care or treatment they gave me, as well as any significant events that occurred, allowing room for additional commentary if they chose to do so. The scope of these responses helped me to reconstruct the hours and days I spent in the emergency room, intensive care unit, and the rehab hospital. These interviews, hospital records, and my own recollections and art work have been combined to form the content of this book which was written during my extensive recovery.

When I first considered writing this book, I was hesitant. I recognized that in order to illuminate my experiences for others I would have to relive the entire harrowing onslaught of sepsis from the mysterious beginning to the acute illness, and through the challenging and lengthy recovery process. This would require prying into horrifying and painful memories etched in my mind, listening to and seeing the suffering of my family, and returning to the hospital to conduct interviews. It would be like reconstructing a physical, mental and spiritual war zone where I was the quarry of an unseen enemy. "Can I do this?" I wondered. "How will it affect my recovery and personal balance?"

These considerations began during my last week in the Wake Med rehab hospital, where I first got the motivation to share my experiences with the world. Since I had limited ability to do anything beyond barely lifting a fork to eat, and very slowly shuffling to the bathroom with a walker and help from a nurse, I had a lot of time to contemplate my existence and to pray, while God inspired me toward this undertaking. I was not strong enough to hold a pen and write sentences and paragraphs. I could only slowly and quietly penetrate my fears and thoughts to begin sketching a mental outline of what had transpired.

There were gaps of time where minutes and hours blended together until fourteen days passed in the ICU, seven more in transitional recovery on the sixth floor, then ten more days on the second floor for rehab. Thirty one days later I was released from the hospital, very weak and fragile and twenty five pounds lighter.

I was extremely happy to go home. There was still a long road to recovery ahead of me. I would go through many challenges, including gall bladder surgery, overcoming pain, anxiety and depression, rebuilding atrophied muscles, and sharpening my cognitive functions back to normal. Weeks and months would pass by while God helped me to become a walking talking miracle.

CHAPTER ONE

THE ONSET

Fall Down Seven Times, Get Up Eight- Japanese Proverb

I turned sixty in May. My tight khakis kept reminding me that I needed to lose weight, so at 5' 11" tall and 236 pounds, I made a commitment to do something about it. The pool at our apartments opened at the end of the month and I began swimming 3-4 times a week, building up to about nine laps before breakfast. I added in more walking, working out with dumbbells, and of course pushups away from the wrong foods.

June was full of sunshine. I felt energetic and positive like I was in tune with myself and the whole world around me. This baby boomer still felt like I had a lot of boom left, so I planned more paintings and drawings, wrote songs, played guitar, and researched ideas and projects on the internet. These busy and pleasant days seemed to accelerate through the calendar like good times do.

July arrived cloaked in mystery. Just after the 4th I began to wonder why I was getting short of breath. It came in little spurts at about 11:00 a.m. every day, but I dismissed it with a cup of coffee and immersed myself in my music and art, working at the computer or running errands. "It must be the air pollution from the freeway that is bothering me," I said, so I wasn't that concerned.

By the end of the first week I began to get a low grade fever at about 99-99.8 degrees. I normally run about 97.5-97.8 degrees when checked at any doctor appointment. I began to have pain around my ears and a headache with pounding sinuses. I took Tylenol and it appeared to back it off for a while, then return the next day. I thought it might be a sinus infection. But, the restricted breathing continued and I now began to encounter pain in my lower right abdomen and lower back. I took more Tylenol and oxycodone for the pain and fever, while my wife Nancy tried hot compresses on my face. Nothing gave me lasting results and my concern grew. Something was wrong but I could not identify it or deal with it.

15 days! From July 4th to the 19th a sleeping infectious monster was slowly waking up. The low grade fever and other symptoms persisted and aggravated me. I became irritable and impatient and was unable to focus on television, movies, or even extended conversations. My attention span kept diminishing and I would fall off to sleep. When my wife and son Dorian returned home from briefly going to the movies for his birthday on Sunday the 19th, they found me bent over in pain, shivering and shaking, first feeling hot then chills. I was rapidly deteriorating and became very worried about my condition. I struggled through that night only sleeping a few hours, then I would sit up or pace back and forth nervously up and down the hallway.

Early Monday morning July 20, 2009, my wife called North Raleigh Primary Care and got a "fit you in" immediate appointment with our doctor, Dr. Joseph M. Micchia, Jr.

Somehow, I slowly managed to shave with shaking hands, take a shower, and get dressed. Urgency dominated the tense atmosphere and I couldn't seem to focus on anything. When I drove to the doctor I could barely keep my mini-van in the lanes. I think that I was on autopilot part of the way. I wasn't judging distances very well and I nearly drove over the curbs pulling into the parking lot. We were both relieved when the van was parked and the engine turned off. I really should have let my wife drive. I began to panic. My internal alarm system was going off and I was rattled.

When I went in to see Dr. Micchia my fever was at 102 degrees, blood pressure 125/71, and pulse at 137. I was dehydrated, sweaty, weak, and becoming dizzy and disoriented. He found blood and white blood cells in my urine which showed signs of significant bacteria. I don't even remember giving the urine sample. He told me in an interview conducted months later that I had "the gray look" that day, like I was ready to collapse and fall apart. I drifted in and out of conversations and felt something overtaking me, nothing like I have ever experienced before. My wife answered medical questions for me, and filled out my paper work. I felt like I was on a raft slowly drifting out to sea away from everyone, even myself. I felt it to the core of my being.

Dr. Micchia told me that I was septic and that I needed to pick a hospital in the next ten minutes. He was familiar with sepsis from his experience at The University of Pittsburgh hospital where he had seen it several times. I didn't know what sepsis was, but I was ready to surrender myself to anyone who could help me. My son Dorian was called, and he left work and came immediately to the doctor's office to help out. Dr. Micchia called ahead to Wake Med Hospital Emergency so that they would know my condition and be ready for me when I arrived. I was willing to go to the hospital, but stubborn about going in an ambulance, so Nancy, Dorian, a nurse, and Dr. Micchia helped me walk out of the back of the office and get into my nearby van. Dr. Micchia's quick and accurate diagnosis of sepsis, and his speedy response in getting me to the Wake Med ER helped to save my life. I am eternally grateful to him.

We were now in the van. My wife drove and my son navigated the streets and signs, and kept an eye on me. The ride to the hospital was a blurred memory of traffic and streets and buildings looking like scrambled and disconnected digital images from a bad cable connection. I remember pulling into the parking area near the emergency room and slowly, cautiously getting out and walking into the hospital. My internal gyroscope was spinning off balance and I could no longer control the escalating panic within me.

We waited for about ten minutes. It seems so much longer when you are beginning to feel desperate and afraid. My son told the staff that I was septic. I was then pre-screened by a nurse who checked my temperature, blood pressure, heart rate and overall appearance. This was conducted in the triage area where preliminary evaluations are done as a process of prioritizing patients based on the severity of their condition. Meanwhile, my wife took care of all the paperwork for patient history, health insurance and admissions. They determined that I needed to go to the emergency room immediately. My wait time was very short compared to many busy city hospitals. My wife, now a worried wreck, accompanied me to the emergency room, while my son waited in another room for half an hour before he was allowed back with me.

I arrived in the emergency room around 10:15 a.m. where I would spend the next 7-8 hours. They conducted several tests which included: EKG's, urinalysis (urine dipstick), x-rays, ultrasounds, CT scans, and a thorough infection/sepsis evaluation. It felt like a continual loop repeated over and over. This was caused by constantly re-evaluating lab reports, and reviewing monitor data and vital sign assessments.

My temperature was 102.1, blood pressure 149/79, and pulse at 129. Positive nitrites were found in urinalysis. My condition showed significant weakness, increasing chills or rigors, fever, flank pain, lightheadedness, dizziness, and pain rated at 10 out of 10. My liver was enlarged and my gall bladder wall had thickened. The diagnosis was defined as acute acalculous cholecystitis (gallbladder inflammation), with concern for systemic infection. I was put on oxygen, placed on intravenous therapy (IV's), and attached to various monitors. The doctors repeatedly asked me questions. I was stubborn, and refused help from my wife and son while they continued questioning me. I insisted on answering them myself. I think that I was impatient and stubborn because I wanted to feel better, but I was getting worse and wanted solutions, not what seemed like an interrogation.

The pain was so overwhelming that morphine in increasing amounts (2mg-4mg) was ineffective, so they tried Fentanyl which gave me some relief. It's a much stronger synthetic opioid for severe pain. At different times they gave me several other medications which included the antibiotics Rocephin, Vancomycin, and Zosyn, acetaminophen for fever and pain, non-steroidal anti-inflammatory drugs (NSAIDS) such as Motrin and Toradol, and later Dilaudid (hydromorphone) which is a potent semi-synthetic opioid, a derivative of morphine.

This seven hour time period was a bewildering gray area for me. My panic had intensified and was starting to overwhelm me, leaving bits and pieces in my memory that didn't seem to connect with any sense of closure or clarity. I believe that the sepsis was causing a rapid deterioration of my mental state as well as my physical condition. I have had a high fever in times past and made it through with Tylenol and cold compresses, but I did not sense a quick fix here. My entire body felt like it was exploding from within, spinning more and more out of balance while my mind battled with obscurity.

Dr. Premakumar described my condition as critical. His addendum notes say that his critical care services were provided to treat and/or prevent clinically significant deterioration that could result in metabolic failure, and that the high probability of sudden and clinically significant deterioration of my condition required his highest level of preparedness to intervene urgently. An ICU bed was then ordered.

At around 6pm they were ready to take me to the medical intensive care unit (MICU) before the next shift change. I do not remember changing into a hospital gown or getting in bed. There were flashes of lights, signs, doorways and faces as they quickly wheeled me down the hall, but I had faded out at this point. All of this time, my wife and son were by my side giving me their love, prayers, and support. They were at the hospital over ten hours that day.

CHAPTER TWO

THE DOWNWARD SPIRAL

It is easy to go down into Hell: night and day, the gates of
dark Death stand wide: but to climb back again, to retrace
one's steps to the upper air-there's the rub, the task
- Virgil

I slowly woke up and didn't know where I was. As the haze
cleared I saw a room that was terribly empty, a sterile void of
unfamiliarity. As I surveyed myself from my thoughts to my
toes, I tried to make sense of things while I began to notice
faint noises and beeps from monitors. I felt things attached to
me like a catheter, IV's, and an oxygen tube clipped to my
nose. I finally noticed the bed I was in, a doorway, shelves,
and a sink and mirror. My mouth was very dry and my tongue felt like a piece of rough leather. I could form words, but
had difficulty speaking them."What am I doing here?"I
feebly spoke aloud. No one answered. I was completely
alone on an island of intensifying pain. As the fog cleared
away, I became more conscious of my whole body feeling
like it was about to explode. This was the kind of pain that
could quickly reduce you into a desperate victim crying for
help, like someone about to drown. I couldn't move. I was a
weak, vulnerable, and petrified soul set adrift in a severe
illness that I could not comprehend. My life was out of

control, and I continually fought to regain my bearings. I groped for a ledge of reality to rest upon, only finding one for a few brief lucid moments then I would drift off into oblivion.

My condition worsened. The descent into the dark abyss of sepsis was rapid, painful, and overwhelming. My entire body was stretched and swollen like an over-inflated rubber raft. My legs felt like huge tree trunks, and my clumsy flipper-like hands were unfinished sculptures intended to be hands, but barely recognizable. My eyes and skin turned a disgusting yellow, and my fever raged sometimes peaking at 104.9, pressing me to the outermost limits of every breath and every thought. My family interviews confirmed many of my observations and feelings. They saw the fear, paranoia, and delirium overwhelm me while I tried to reach out to them with wilted hands or force words with a dark shriveled prune-like tongue. I was in and out of consciousness and was convinced that I wasn't going to make it to the next day. Time was a lost dimension for me. I had no idea what day or hour it was. I stared at the large round clock on the wall and thought it was jumping from 10pm to 4am in a few moments. I had times when I insisted that I saw the clock move ahead one minute to 10:31 and then go backwards to 10:30. This really got to me. It seemed like I was in my own time zone.

Doctors and nurses came into the room and invaded my distorted space. "Who are these people?" I said cautiously. "What is happening to me?" I don't remember their exact responses, but the tone was reassuring. They annoyed me with constant questions. "What is your name?" "What year is it?" "What month and day is it?" I got my name and the year right, but that was about all. I reacted to them as if they were jailers trying to keep me in the room and interrogate me.

Everyone looked orange as I squinted through my tired yellow eyes, and the room had a light blue fuzzy haze covering every shape. I felt trapped and miserable. I had begun to cascade into severe sepsis, fighting a massive infection spreading in my bloodstream.

During my first few days in the ICU I had IV's in both hands, a blood pressure sleeve on my left arm and a small sensor clip on one finger that went to monitors, and a oxygen tube in my nose(nasal cannula). I heard a pump running and felt something squeezing the calf muscles of my lower legs. This was a sequential compression device (SCD) designed to improve circulation and to avoid clot formation or deep vein thrombosis where blood tends to pool in the calf area of the lower leg. The SCD consists of an air pump connected to a sleeve by a series of air tubes. The sleeve is placed around a patient's leg. Venous return is improved by intermittently forcing air in sequence into different parts of the sleeve. I know it was necessary, but I found it to be very annoying and added it to my list of things that disturbed my peace and quiet.

When it was time to use the bed pan I panicked. I cringed at the thought of it. It took several people to move me, usually two very patient male nurses and one or both of my sons when they were available. I came into the hospital at around 236 pounds, add in the edema weight and I probably weighed between 240-245 pounds. Many times they needed four people to do it. I could not stand to be moved or touched because the pain was so intense, even morphine didn't calm it so they gave me a more potent drug called Fentanyl. I was swollen and very heavy, and my four hernia surgeries from years past were strained to the limit from the entire bowel movement process. I would groan and cry out loudly until it was over, and then I was left exhausted, withered, and speechless. I couldn't use a urine cup because my entire rectal/scrotal area was swollen several times larger than normal. Soon after this, catheters were implemented, one for urine, and a few days later another for fecal management. The anal catheter installation, removal, and re-installation brought me to tears, and there was nothing I could do about it. This was more than I could bear.

My confinement became magnified by the increasing number of attachments to my body, and the other devices in the ICU. They took me to Radiology where a cholecystostomy was performed. They made an incision through the abdomen and installed a tube placed in the gallbladder which drained dark greenish brown bile into a collection bag. The cholecystostomy tube (gallbladder tube) was very uncomfortable. I had a lot of pain in my right side. To make things worse, this initial installation of the gallbladder tube didn't function properly, so the tube had to be replaced in Radiology a few days later. A liver biopsy was also done.

My fever would fluctuate from hour to hour and day to day from 99.9 to 100.3, to 102.1, to 103.0, and sometimes back to 99.6 degrees. My wife, who was next to me most of the time, saw my temperature peak once at 104.9 and yelled for a nurse. That is when they decided to bring in a cooling blanket to place underneath me to lower and stabilize my body temperature. This was difficult to do because of the severe pain I felt when they tried to move me. The blanket was connected to cables and hoses that went to a big circulating pump that had a temperature monitor for the water. They also installed a rectal thermometer in me.

Next, a peripherally inserted central catheter (PICC) was installed on my arm which allowed intravenous access for a prolonged period of time, such as the extended antibiotic therapy that I received. The PICC line is a thin flexible tube inserted into a vein, usually in the bend of your arm. It is longer, more stable and secured in place and can reduce irritation or damage to the blood vessels in your arms from multiple blood draws and IV insertions. You can receive fluids, blood transfusions, nutrition and medications, and also use it for obtaining blood for laboratory tests. I received red blood cells, pain medications, nutrition and antibiotics. I also received an IV NAC with acetylcysteine which is used for acetaminophen overdose.

All of these attachments and strange devices frustrated me and contributed to my anxiety, disorientation, and stress, yet they were necessary for my survival. I was a weak vulnerable prisoner in the ICU that felt trapped and desperate. Several days had now passed since I entered the ICU, and I wasn't feeling any better. The cascade of sepsis evolved. My illness continued to induce feelings of paranoia, fear, and distrust toward the doctors and nurses. Voices of my family and the hospital staff would seem distant and reverberate as if they were talking inside a tunnel or through a long hollow tube. I began to worry about dying. After being in the ICU for over a week I overheard a doctor telling my wife and son that if my condition did not improve in the next 24-48 hours, they would lose me. This put me on edge. I felt like my entire life was hanging by a thread.

I was convinced that calling the rest of my family meant that I was going to die very soon. I wanted to break out of this prison, tear down the sides of the bed, and walk out of the ICU and out the front door of the hospital. Then, I would run down the street to the freeway and make my way home. These thoughts prevailed as I became more and more frustrated in my confinement. I hated the PICC attached to my arm. I was exhausted from struggling with pain in my body and disorientation in my mind.

I planned my escape. Late that night about 4am, I waited until I was alone. As soon as the nurse left the room I dislodged the oxygen tube in my nose, ripped the PICC out of my arm and pulled back the bloody blanket to begin my escape to freedom. I urged myself forward, but I could not move my legs. My face became frozen in awe as I looked at two huge fleshy tree trunks that were swollen to twice their normal size from the sepsis. I tried again even harder, but still could not move, yet alone stand up and walk. My swollen fingers and hands could barely grab the side of the bed. They looked like medical exam gloves expanded out of proportion with an air pump. I cried in despair. I was defeated and I was going nowhere. I wanted to crawl inside myself somewhere and hide from everything. "I will never leave here," I said to myself. That bewildered moment became etched in my memory as I shuddered at thoughts of my demise. There was no escape, "what was I thinking?"

Within minutes nurses frantically came to my rescue, saving me from myself and my own distorted paranoia and delirium. Soon a new central line was attached to me, but this time in my neck, and the oxygen tube was returned to my nose. I was not aware that they did this because I was fading in and out of consciousness. I am surprised that they didn't put restraints on my hands. The next time I woke up and reconnected with reality, the doctors and nurses explained to me just what had happened, and how that could have been my last night in the hospital and my last day on earth.

The doctor's reports confirmed the escalating sepsis as it continued to rage like a California wildfire inside of me. They also estimated and explained the possible causes of my mental state. A vast array of tests were implemented which gave the doctors and nurses continual feedback about my condition. They included: CT scans, MRI's, ultrasounds, liver biopsy, a copper test for Wilson's disease, and lab reports for blood and urinalysis, as well as monitoring bile collected through my cholecystostomy tube attached to my gallbladder. They also checked my temperature, heart rate, breathing, oxygen level, fluids, overall appearance and mental acuity. The CT scans revealed a very small non-obstructive kidney stone which was not considered a problem, and a recent tick bite was evaluated by disease control which checked out fine after test results returned. My white blood cell count was normal.

Dr. Whitt from Gastroenterology examined me and determined that my condition was consistent with biliary sepsis, with concern for a possible duct stone. He described my condition as worsening with jaundice, delirium and encephalopathy. Dr. Rutherford came in for surgery consultation to evaluate the need for gallbladder intervention. His first comments were that it was an unclear clinical scenario with questionable gallbladder findings, and he wanted to wait for further medical consultations and results beyond the evident increased liver tests and the nitrites and bacteria found in urinalysis. Both of these doctors were very kind and patient with me.

I had already met sepsis criteria with tachycardia (fast heart rate), tachypnea (rapid breathing), fever, rigors, organ defects (altered liver and kidney function), and an abnormal heart rhythm (asymptomatic junctional rhythm) which they closely monitored. My situation intensified, and I became acutely ill and was on continual fluid resuscitation. The working diagnosis was sepsis presumed secondary to acalculous cholecystitis (inflammation of the gallbladder). My gallbladder wall had thickened. My whole body inflammatory state caused a distended abdomen and edema of the scrotal area and bilateral lower extremities. The bacterial infection over-stimulated my immune system (the chemical signals went out of control) setting off a cascade of inflammatory and abnormal clotting responses inside my blood vessels. I was anemic and had thrombocytopenia (low blood platelet count) as well as hypertension with blood pressure in the 140's to 150's. My bilirubin count peaked at 13.0. I had acute hepatic injury with coagulopathy (blood clotting problems) and finally acute liver failure and acute renal failure, followed by multifactorial encephalopathy (brain dysfunction caused by infection, organ failure, and other disorders). The vicious cycle of inflammation and coagulation intensified the sepsis cascade.

INFECTION → SIRS → SEPSIS → SEVERE SEP-
SIS/SEPTIC SHOCK → DEATH

My fight with internal terror continued as I grew closer and
closer to death. I now had severe sepsis with multiple organ
failure, with possible hepatic (liver) or anoxic (oxygen deficient) encephalopathy which brought about an altered mental
state. I had a very impaired attention span, and required
repeated verbal cues to stay on task during a conversation. I
was unable to complete sentences and refused to communicate with some doctors. I was anxious, lethargic, and confused. My delirium included flights of ideas, confabulations
(confusing imagination with memory and facts), grandiosity,
and inappropriate laughter. I would easily go off on tangents,
which may have been intensified by pain killers such as
morphine or Fentanyl or other medications. I was caught in
an emotional storm, and I felt like I was nearing death as the
waves of pain and delirium came crashing down on me.

When you are grasping for any thread of hope, and the pain
and suffering is more than you can bear, and your innermost
being is preparing to surrender to the next place; you are near
death. You know. You just know. "Don't bury me here," I
told my wife. I made my sons promise to send me home to
Ohio, my birthplace and where I grew up. At this point I
told my wife:"I'm ready to go." I held her hand while the
tears clouded my eyes and I prepared to say goodbye. I felt
myself sinking into oblivion. There were shadows of darkness permeating the air around me. My wife boldly replied:"You're not going anywhere!" With great determination
and insistence she commanded that I not go, but stay with
her. Her brave words, faithful prayers, and heart beating in

unison with mine brought me a lifeline which I held onto during my weakest moments. I was at peace and ready to make my journey into the next realm, but God chose to take me back from the edge of darkness and continue my life here. A divine intervention had begun.

I wrote a song about this time period in the ICU. It describes my desperation, suffering, imprisonment, and alienation as well as glimmers of hope in the midst of the agony and delirium of sepsis.

WHERE AM I?   Gary Black, 2009

I'm inside looking out.
They can't hear me if I shout.
It's a prison that I'm in, Where Am I?
All the shapes before my eyes…
Is it the devil in disguise?
It's a prison that I'm in, Where Am I?
I hear voices all around,
But I don't recognize a sound.
It's a prison that I'm in, Where Am I?
The pain is everywhere,
And it's more than I can bear.
It's a prison that I'm in, Where Am I?

I don't want to be touched.
I don't know where I am,
Just leave me alone.
Let me out of this place,
so I can call someone,

And they can come and take me home,
Where Am I?

It feels like outer space,
when you don't recognize a face.
It's a prison that I'm in, Where Am I?
The darkness fell on me,
A piano from the sky,
It's a prison that I'm in, Where Am I?
Somehow through it all,
I can see you on the wall.
It's a prison that I'm in, Where Am I?
It's love that lifted me,
the only thing that set me free,
from the prison that I'm in, Where Am I?

I don't want to be touched.
I don't know where I am,
Just leave me alone.
Let me out of this place,
so I can call someone,
And they can come and take me home,
Where Am I?

Time is slowly slipping by me,
And all these things just seem to try me,
And I don't feel like I am here,
No I don't feel like I am here,
Where Am I?

I don't want to be touched.
I don't know where I am,

Just leave me alone.
Let me out of this place,
So I can call someone,
And they can come and take me home,
Where Am I? Where Am I? Where Am I?

CHAPTER THREE

DREAMS AND DELIRIUM

Long is the way and hard, that out of hell leads up to
light. - John Milton

My Dreams and Delirium

You have stretched my face with fear,
and plunged my soul to murky depths,
where I stumbled in the dark.

I was a strong tree standing in a field,
until the torrent of rain and hail
stripped me of my bark.

With arms outstretched to heaven,
I waited to be delivered,
"God help me" was what I cried.

I drifted into dreams and delirium,
those tangents of the unknown,
"Was I awake or had I died?"

I remember the rampage through my thoughts,
and the raging fire in my body,
while in my prison of affliction.

The darkness and the light came and went
in the depths of my departures,
Those veiled mysterious moments, were they truth or fiction?

Many of the situations that I have described to you about the ICU took on a whole new meaning and dimension for me in my dreams and delirium. My sedated sleep was transformed into mindscapes and emotional storms that included episodes of horror, fear, paranoia, flights of imagination and religious experiences like I have never had in my entire life. All of the spaces of time in between tests and while my family was visiting became periods of deep sleep, deeper and farther from the fierce reality of the ICU room where I transformed into altered mental states that I perceived as reality. In some cases, my delirium became a spiritual awakening and a comfort to my soul.

I have depicted several of these events in my drawings which are accurate renditions of what I saw and remembered while in the ICU. I still remember most of the episodes clearly, and with details that sometimes come back to haunt me. The situations I found myself in at the time felt completely real, and sometimes I did not feel as though I could escape out of them back to some sense of tangible reality. At times it felt like my altered world held a power over me, and would not let me come back no matter how hard I resisted and cried out. I would feel completely helpless and alone, like someone lost in a cave without even a match and a candle. There was a constant crossing back and forth over the border of reality into a distorted view of the room I was in and the people I saw or spoke with. When I woke up I would feel joy and peace seeing my family by my bedside, but it was easy to see their deep concern and worry that they tried to hide behind their forced smiles and hopeful eyes. Many times I thought it would be the last time I would see them. My self–portraits attempt to capture my innermost feelings of raw fear, anguish and depression, but also hope and peace. Months and months later the dreams and episodes are still with me and not forgotten. I have had more dreams while writing this story.

Medical professionals have described my experiences as possible ICU psychosis brought upon by several contributing factors in my strange environment such as sleep disruption, unfamiliar people, uncomfortable procedures, and constant noises inherent in the ICU, as well as the effects of medications and acute illness. My altered mental state has been described as multifactorial encephalopathy with possibilities of hepatic and/or anoxic influences. This can be precipitated by the lack of oxygen to the brain, high bilirubin count in the liver, and opiate and synthetic opiod pain killers. The end result is delirium.

Some of the diagnostic terms used to describe my condition included: encephalopathy, psychosis, hallucinations, delusions, delirium, and ICU psychosis (environmental), all contributing to the spectrum of experiences that I endured.

Encephalopathy generally refers to dysfunction of the brain, and in my case caused by the systemic illness of sepsis, related metabolic disorders, organ failure, and oxygen deficiency resulting in an altered mental state. Symptoms can include changes in behavior and personality, lethargy, inability to concentrate, confusion, disorientation, and loss of cognitive functions.

Psychosis is an abnormal mental condition, a loss of contact with reality which may include hallucinations, delusions, personality changes and thought disorders. It may be characterized as a distorted or nonexistent sense of objective reality. I suffered with many of these symptoms during my battle with sepsis. I had hallucinations with distorted sensory experiences that appeared to be real perceptions, and delusions where I formed unshakable and irrational beliefs in something untrue, defying normal reasoning. I also experienced ICU psychosis. I developed anxiety, restlessness and irritation which were influenced by inherent factors of the ICU environment. The contributing factors included frequent interruptions, sleep deprivation or disruption, noises and equipment operating, unfamiliar people, and uncomfortable procedures, all occurring in an unfamiliar setting.

Delirium entered the picture or diagnosis as a fluctuating disturbance of mental function with a set of symptoms caused by a chemical and/or disease process. These symptoms included disturbance of consciousness, change in cognition, disorientation and confusion resulting in possible hallucinations, delusions, and a dream-like state. There may also be abrupt mood changes, paranoia, poor attention span, and impaired short term memory and recall. I experienced most of these symptoms. This acute and debilitating disorder developed into a dramatic altered mental state that left me feeling lost, helpless, afraid, and isolated. The incendiary and overlapping symptoms of the dream/delirium amalgam defied reality and challenged the very core of my being. I was given

Haldol (Haloperidol) which is a high potency antipsychotic drug used for the treatment of acute psychosis and acute delirium.

The language of imagery in dreams unfolded my subjective experiences of imaginary shapes, colors, sounds, voices, thoughts, and sensations during my sleep. I have many memories of my experiences ranging from the real to the surreal with episodes that were inspiring, frightening, symbolic, and meaningful.

Arthur Schopenhauer said: "A dream is short lasting psychosis, and a psychosis is a long lasting dream." Sigmund Freud wrote: "A dream then, is a psychosis." (Wikipedia Encyclopedia, 2010).These are interesting descriptions to think about. My dreams provided me with a means of escape from a painful and terrifying existence in the ICU where I struggled against a barrage of illness. But, many of the escapes left me stranded on an island of confusion, delusion, and even hallucination. The dreams were permeated with delirium where I coped with perceived threats and confrontations with darkness, purgatory, and impending death. I side stepped one stressful reality and found myself in another distorted restructured one filled with anxiety, stress, and entrapment. There were brief times where flights of imagination gave me some relief and renewal, but most of my dreams and delirium became an internal war in the surreal, asleep from one world and awake in another. I still remember them and have had recurrences months later. I have depicted some of them in my art work in Chapter 10.

From my perspective, the sum of all of these events was a very significant part of the overwhelming illness. It did not go away. I still remember a vast amount of occurrences, and I feel it in my spirit and watch it unfold in my art work. So, while doctors treated my acute physical illness for the most part, and my exhibited delirium with the antipsychotic Haldol, my spirit was soaring near death, through purgatory, and even down the hall from my room. Now, I am reporting back to you from journeys of mind and spirit.

The Doctor/Nurse Conspiracy

As my illness progressed I became paranoid, feeding my fear with irrational beliefs and distrust. I actually believed that the doctors and nurses were devious and had constructed a secret web of conspiracy to keep me in the hospital. They were all jailers holding me captive in a bed of continual misery and suffering. I didn't trust anyone. I questioned every move they made. I would ask everyone to leave the room except for my two sons, and then I would ask them if these people around me were "ok". If they did not say something was alright, I would not cooperate.

"Someone changed the room around to fool me", I said. People, computers, monitors, windows, and doors kept changing positions from the day before, or perhaps it was a few hours before, and I woke up confused about it. The walls and cupboards seemed to be relocated in different places, and I thought it was done intentionally. I also thought that someone kept moving the hands on the big round clock on the wall. They were plotting against me to keep me confused about what day it was or what time it was. "Who are these people?" I said firmly and suspiciously. "What are they doing to me?" I began to worry that I would never leave this place. I kept staring at the wall clock wondering, "How much time do I have?" I felt trapped, depressed, and isolated and wanted to get out of there. This led up to the night I ripped out the IV's and oxygen tube in a failed escape attempt that almost killed me.

Only my family could help me reconnect with reality and accept help from the doctors and nurses as they tried to accomplish their daily routines. My suspicions were not well founded or logical. I was looking through the distorted lenses of an acute illness that was overtaking me. The doctors and nurses were there to help me, not to conspire against me in the ICU. Actually, they were soft spoken, kind, and patient with good intentions toward reviving my health.

The Secret Underground

I was convinced that I was trapped inside an evil realm of illegal activities going on in the hospital. This secret underground was carefully disguised. The doctors, nurses and hospital staff had another business hidden within the daily hospital curriculum. They controlled all of the patients and sold drugs and artificial enhancements for profit. They would never let you leave once you entered their evil domain. I felt like I had no one to talk to about it. I could not trust anyone. Who would believe me? My paranoia had no boundaries, and now included the entire hospital.

I was awake then asleep, awake then into a deeper sleep, over and over until I could no longer distinguish between the two states. I looked asleep, but struggled in twilight. This dimension felt like an artificial reality composed of a maze of rooms full of changing wall panels, shelves and cupboards, computer screens, faded images, and strange people smiling at me while they worked. It seemed like a business center or office building with people talking on phones and walking back and forth. Most of them ignored me. The shifts seemed to change often and I saw no familiar faces. I tried to talk to them, but they smiled and hurried past my bed without responding. There was a drug boss dressed in an expensive gray suit with several other workers who distributed products. He had set up a download industry with sales offering encoded discs for items and services throughout the hospital. My wife told me that at one point of grandiosity I claimed to be the drug leader, which was of course untrue.

There would be no peace or quiet for your mind and body until you paid them over the phone with a credit card for special credits that you used for illegal items such as "special services" and drugs called "joy powders". I remember constantly trying to buy "time spaces" for total quiet so that I could rest, and always being hungry and thirsty with nothing available to eat or drink. I was extremely frustrated, helpless, and confused. I could not escape this evil manipulating realm. I wanted out so badly. Then, in a sudden shift of consciousness, I would wake up to the humming and beeping equipment in the ICU.

The Demented Nurses

In the first dream I was taken to a building out on a rural farm. The room was full of huge, round metal tubs that looked similar to the inside of commercial washing machines. They were full of ice cold water. There were several nurses. They appeared fat, mean, and demented. They were wearing nurse's dresses, aprons, and hats. Their hair was unkempt and they looked scary, like weird nurses abusing and taunting patients in a horror movie about some psycho ward in an old hospital, starring Florence Nightingale's imaginary deranged sisters. They stared at me with cruel and wicked eyes, and talked about fertility of cows and themselves. I wanted to get away from them.

They had a leather harness around my chest and over my shoulders. I was completely naked and the water in the tank was so cold that I began to shiver and shake. They laughed and grinned while they lowered me into the tank with a gear and pulley system. One nurse thoroughly enjoyed shoving the lever up and down as I hung there paralyzed in fear. I begged them to release me and they just laughed. My mouth was very dry, but they refused to give me a drink. I feared that the water in the tank might not be clean enough to drink, so there I was surrounded by water and still thirsty.

The second time I had the dream with the water tanks, I found myself hidden away in the basement of the hospital. The walls were dark and made of concrete block. There were stairs going down to the tanks with a locked gate at the top. The demented nurses had thrown me over the railing at the top of the wall into one of the tanks, and then stood there glaring at me with evil grins and laughing. They had another guy with them that they were ready to throw into one of the other tanks. He was yelling and looked terrified. In both dreams I was too weak to pull myself up out of the water tanks, and I remained at the mercy of the crazed nurses. I would slowly wake up to the noises in the ICU where I found myself lying on a cooling blanket used to reduce my fever and stabilize my body temperature.

The House in the Woods

Although I sing, play guitar and write songs, in this dream I was a spectator watching someone else struggle and suffer with their music. I was invited by an eccentric guy who was working on some songs at a recording studio in the back of a house in a remote area of Florida. We drove there in his big white SUV, going off the main highway, down some secondary roads, and then on to unpaved sand roads to get there. The dark brown wood sided house was partially hidden by a lot of ferns and palm trees, and there were no other houses nearby. The studio was in the back of the house. It had a huge, lightly tinted window looking out at the driveway, and a room full of musical equipment. He had his own engineer and several sensuous female backup singers wearing mini-skirts.

He was an older, very thin pale man, with long straight blonde hair. He looked aged and worn out, and struggled with his health. He wore a nose clip for oxygen and had an IV hooked up to one arm. A sexy nurse accompanied him and watched the nearby monitors. He had a very good voice, but it was all he could do to get through one song, then he was out of breath and had to sit down and recover for a while. He was trying so hard and I felt compassion for him. It was difficult to watch. His mind was on his music and he didn't talk with me or ask for any comments about the songs. I thought that was odd, considering that he brought me here and then treated me like a stranger.

In between recordings I sat in a dimly lit lounge, sometimes for hours. The walls were painted black, the carpet was dark purple, and the couches were black leather. The atmosphere felt strange, moody and uncomfortable. I would talk with the backup singers who were very bored waiting around to do small vocal parts. I told them I wanted to leave. They told me that no one was allowed to leave, and that we were locked in. I began to panic and felt trapped. Fortunately, about this time I woke up in the ICU feeling very relieved that I had escaped the house in the woods.

The Old Warehouse

I found myself in an old warehouse in Amsterdam. It was made of faded brown and reddish brown bricks and had an abundance of windows covered with years of moisture and dust. The entrance had a huge weathered wood door that led to abandoned offices, where I could faintly see a canal and a bridge through one of the dirty windows. There were dust covered chairs and desks and a set of double doors that brought me into the warehouse. This area was cleaner and had several platforms, steps, and partitioned rooms that may have been different workshops at one time. There was a large multi-tiered stage at the very back of the massive room.

There was a collection of old foreign guitar amplifiers in the rooms and all over different levels of the big stage area. These amplifiers looked strange, with metal grills and metal cabinets looking like aged porcelain in color. At first I thought they were heating or cooling devices, but after closer inspection I could see the speakers behind the grills and control knobs on the back. I found out that they were collector's amps made in Holland and Germany in the late 40's and 50's. People prized these tube amps and cherished them for their unique tonal qualities.

I met some local people that played jazz with them. They were practicing in the back of the warehouse up on the high tiers of the stage. I played guitar with them in an abstract jam session, where little was said between us, yet we spoke the language of music to each other in our notes. When I woke up again in the ICU, I was startled by the noise coming from the metal encased pump unit at the foot of my bed, as it circulated water through the cooling blanket underneath me.

The Black Room/Purgatory

My most distinct dreams, deliriums, or spiritual travels took place in the black room I call Purgatory, where I fought for my own soul, and examined my motivations and values in life.

In the first episode I thought that I had inherited part of an estate from someone in Colorado. I was invited to a restaurant somewhere near Colorado Springs where recipients were summoned to receive their portion of the inheritance. After entering the restaurant, and passing by shelves with gourmet wines, cheeses, and hand-painted decorative items, I was directed to a particular door in the back of the place. I opened the door, stepped in, and suddenly found myself locked in a pitch black room with no way out. There were several rooms actually, and they were full of impatient, sick, and unhappy people who complained that when they accepted their portion of the inheritance they became ill and possessed by it somehow. Some were envious about what the others claimed to have, <u>yet you couldn't see anything in the dark.</u> This terrified me all the way down to my bones and my spirit. It was a Purgatory full of wandering souls trying to find their way out. I heard voices muttering and complaining while they were self-absorbed in their own misery. They did not talk to me. I used the voices and utterances to help step around them. Some just stood there, while others were crouched on the floor. I tapped the metal walls for hours, looking for a way out, which I finally found. I saw a tiny light beaming in the distance coming from a narrow rectangular window on what appeared to be a door. There was a ramp going up to this steel door with a window full of light. I pulled very hard. It opened and I squeezed through the partially opened door to make my escape. As I left, I paused for a brief moment and looked back at a room full of people with sad sunken eyes, crying and moaning in desperation. I quickly closed the door to this horrible dark room of lamentation. I awakened to the beeping monitors in the ICU.

The second episode was very similar to the first, but it was much more intense and terrifying. I was in a deep sleep I thought, but I found myself in the black room again. Cold and dark it was, like a damp basement full of stale air, smelling like soiled sweaty clothing and moist bricks and concrete. The fear and darkness made my soul shiver. My anxiety began to torture me in this empty void. Was I dead or in Purgatory?

I began to hear heavy breathing, like anxious sighs at a funeral. A few voices came within range, and they were mumbling and crying with a sorrowful tone. I stumbled around the room bumping into several people as I tried to find a way out. Once again, they were complaining about their portion of the inheritance and the unfair manner of which it was distributed. Some thought they were to receive millions and were only given worthless vague items.

There was a terrible vibe to this room. I felt so lost, and my only thought was to find a way out of there. The sad drone of the people banished in this darkness pulled at me like death whispering in my ears. I knew that if I stayed here, I would be consumed by this place and never return. This time it seemed like days not hours that I searched frantically through several of these rooms, tapping the walls and trying to hear my way around. No one even spoke to me. Everyone was caught up in their own despair.

Again, I saw a tiny light coming from a narrow window on a huge steel door. I made my way onto a walkway and came up to it. I felt around and found a handle which I pushed down and opened the door. Again, I squeezed out through the partially opened door. I looked back and saw more depressed and hopeless faces, but this time, there were taunting devilish figures creeping around too. I swiftly slammed the door behind me and walked into the light, finding myself back in the ICU again.

I went back to the black Purgatory room several times. In each journey I felt like I was near death and trapped in a dark room with lamenting lost souls, and each time I found the light from the small window on the door and made my way out. I thought that on the conscious surface I was fighting death physically, while my mind and spirit struggled through Purgatory shaking the very foundation of my being.

These episodes in the ICU felt like an eternity. Minutes could have been hours, and hours could have been days while I journeyed through my illness. The ICU became my safe harbor to return to after crossing back and forth through the gateway to darkness. Every time I saw the bright light and followed it, I escaped Purgatory and death. These journeys occurred during the time that one of the doctors told my wife that if I didn't improve in the next 24-48 hours, they would lose me.

The end was near, and I could feel it pulling me like a rip tide out into an ocean of oblivion. Was it a dream or delirium? It felt real to me, and it still does. I have had several enlightening recurrences. I believe that I had true spiritual experiences and awakenings that have helped bring about changes in my life. I visited the edge of death and darkness and grew in the light.

CHAPTER FOUR

THE TURNING POINT

My grace is sufficient for thee: for my strength is made perfect in weakness - II Corinthians 12:9

It was my last four days in the ICU, but I didn't know that. I thought I was dying. God truly blessed and guided the doctors who cared for me, and combined with his divine presence around me, I began to recover. My near death experiences took me down into a deep, dark Purgatory, and even for a walk outside of myself down the hall. Skirting near death was exhausting, yet revealing and enlightening. Part of me had prepared for death and departure while the other part reached for the light. My dreams and delirium were crystallized in my memory while inner peace began to spring up within me. A multiple healing process of body, mind, and spirit had begun. I was summoned to the light, and I felt a divine presence in the ICU. In tiny, but noticeable increments, I began to stabilize and recover. Dr. Whitt said to me, "You're healing yourself!" I replied, "No, God is doing it!"

Nancy asked me to get my mind off of any negative dreams and delirium and focus on God. When I did that I felt better. I remembered an old church hymn where the chorus says: "Love lifted me", and I thought, that's what God is doing. He is lifting me up with his light and his love, (that light I followed out of the dark Purgatory). So I started singing it over and over, "Love lifted me." I told the nurses, "Love lifted me!" When my family visited I sang to them, "Love lifted me!" You know, it revived my spirit and renewed my hope. I felt it in the air, that divine presence radiating throughout the room. My wife Nancy, two sons Dorian and Adrian, daughter-in-law Kari, two sisters Cindy and Kathy, and niece Lyla and her husband Joshua surrounded me with their loving support and prayers which brought me positive injections not found in my IV's. They held my hand often, and told me over and over "You're going to get better." My sons and wife brought me vitamin drinks and pleaded and encouraged me to drink them, even though I struggled to use a straw, to swallow, or to speak. They were persistent, dedicated, and full of kindness and compassion. What a great family!

At one point, I found myself walking down the hall outside the ICU, looking at the nurse's station and peering into various rooms with patients lying in their beds. I wasn't physically distressed in any way, and I moved around freely. My steps felt light and airy, and I didn't feel the floor beneath my feet. I had a complete sense of freedom from my illness and felt fine. I told my wife about it, and she told me that I never left the bed, and that I could not sit up or even hold a drink in my swollen hands, yet alone get out of bed or stand up. But, I did leave the bed. My spirit and soul left my pain ridden body behind for a while, and I still remember that peaceful walk.

My sister Cindy was asked to go to the hospital and sit with me, because my wife was exhausted and resting from spending so many hours at my bedside. My niece's husband quickly took her over to the hospital from her hotel.

She arrived a little early, just before visiting hours, but they let her in my room. She sat alone in the corner of the room, deeply praying for me. The lights were down low, and everything was very quiet. She felt a peaceful, glowing presence come into the room. At first she thought it might be a nurse, but when she looked up no one was there. This distinct radiating presence conveyed a feeling of peace, like an invisible spiritual glow you could sense but not see. She said it was stronger over by my bed and the nearby sink and mirror, and it made her feel like everything would be fine. I had sensed moments like this too, where there was a soothing presence in the room, but when an actual nurse or doctor would enter the room, it disappeared. I thought it was the divine presence of God or his emissaries watching over me. My sister said that the presence was overwhelming and made the rectangular room appear full and round with peace emanating everywhere. She did not sense anything negative about it, only peace and assurance that everything was going to be alright. Even Dr. Rutherford, my surgeon, told me once, "Someone up there is looking out for you!" I laid there like a wounded warrior returning to consciousness after a monumental battle with a devastating enemy. My turning point had arrived and I began to recover from the edge of death. I was surviving sepsis.

The day finally came when they released me from the ICU. I had no consciousness of time and did not realize that 14 days had gone by. They pushed my bed down the hall and stopped near some windows to give me a look. "Is that outside?" I asked. "Yes it is", the nurse replied. I gazed in amazement. It was a soft purple morning with a yellow haze. The buildings were not recognizable. At first I thought I saw pyramids in Egypt floating on a mirage of yellow beige sand. It looked like another world. I had been isolated and disconnected long enough to have hours, days, and weeks blend together into a collage I could not easily untangle. When the doctor back in the ICU gave me 24-48 hours to improve or die, it hit me very hard. I was devastated by it and constantly asked the doctors and nurses, "Am I going to make it?" I perseverated on this for several days. I was now on the way to the 6th floor to begin my transition into recovery. I was relieved to survive the ICU, but more challenges were ahead of me.

I arrived at my room on the 6th floor "deconditioned", meaning weak, out of shape, and unable to do many activities. You could simply say that I was beat up and out of it. I could not walk or do much of anything. I could barely lift a spoon or hold a straw for a drink. I could not get out of bed to go to the bathroom, so nurses helped me slowly get up and get seated on a toilet chair unit, while the rest of the time I wore adult diapers. The nurses also bathed me. This was refreshing, but sometimes it was difficult because I seemed to have pain everywhere, and was very sensitive about being touched. The catheters were gone, but I still had the gallbladder tube going out of my side into a drain bag. I continued to take antibiotics, and I was so exhausted that I slept most of the time.

My compassionate and energetic hospitalist, Dr. Alisha Benner described my condition as being very scared, weak, and vulnerable. She was concerned about my circular thinking, and my perseverating on various topics, especially constantly asking, "Am I going to make it?" She said that I was friendly and did a lot of talking as a coping mechanism to help relate to a sense of normalcy. I think that I was still struggling with the effects of encephalopathy and altered cognitive functions. Dr. Benner was very kind, patient and concerned about my progress. She even made me a peanut butter sandwich which I asked for constantly, but when I finally got it I could only manage to eat one or two bites of it. In her interview, she summarized by saying that doctors and nurses need to realize that when a patient is in the hospital, they are at their weakest frail condition, and need special help. She implemented this in the care she gave me.

Susan, one of my other nurses, was also very kind and patient with all of the details of maintaining my care, which included helping me in and out of bed, and in and out of a nearby chair to build my strength. She reheated my food if I was tired and could not eat, opened drinks and straws and placed them within reach, and adjusted my pillows. She also spent a lot of time talking with me, which I greatly appreciated. She did all the little things to make life easier.

My appetite returned and I began to eat. I slowly, cautiously lifted food to my mouth and tried to balance small drinks in my shaky weak hands. I was so excited when I got my first breakfast (which I selected from the menu). I had apple juice, excellent coffee, scrambled eggs, pancakes, grits and apple pieces. I couldn't eat it all, but it was a thrill to even look at. My other meals were actually quite good, but the most exciting moments came when my wife showed up with an ice cold, sinfully delicious chocolate milk shake. There is nothing that competes with that after you have been confined all day in a hospital bed.

My wife filled the shelves in my room with bread, peanut butter (my favorite), jam, bottles of spring water, high protein energy bars, vitamin drinks, and yogurts that the nurses kept in a refrigerator. On the weekend she would cook some of my favorite foods and bring them to my room. I was excited when she brought the meals, but sometimes I didn't eat them. Other times, I was content with just a cafeteria cheeseburger.

I was also very comforted with all of the get well cards that covered the bathroom door and the family photos on a window of another door. The cards and photos helped to dispel the emptiness that I felt from being alone in a hospital room, and kept me connected with family and friends.

The lens slowly turned for me as my life began to come back into focus. Six days had passed on the 6th floor as I left behind the blurred massive distortion of severe sepsis, and began to piece together tiny increments of tangible reality as I grappled toward recovery. The next stage of my recovery was about to begin. I would be going to the Wake Med Rehab hospital which was interconnected to the main hospital.

CHAPTER FIVE

THE REHAB HOSPITAL

The more serious the illness, the more important it is for
you to fight back, mobilizing all your resources-spiritual,
emotional, intellectual, physical. - Norman Cousins

After stabilizing on the 6th floor, I was carefully evaluated.
They determined that I was a good candidate for admission
to a comprehensive inpatient rehabilitation program. Now, I
was taken to the 2nd floor and placed in state of the art rehab
at the two-story, 78 bed WakeMed Rehab hospital. Here I
participated in a recovery program with a daily schedule of a
minimum of three hours of physical, occupational, nursing,
and speech therapy services. I was reevaluated to determine
goals and a treatment program designed to help me return to
as normal a life as possible. I had a clinical case manager
who was the team leader and coordinator of all treatments
implemented by the members of the team, which included: a
specialized rehab nurse, dietician, physical therapist, occupational therapist, speech pathologist, neuropsychologist, rehab
specialty physician, physician's assistant, and a primary
doctor. These people who specialize in rehab have both
clinical qualifications, and unique abilities to be patient,
communicate, and motivate you to reach your goals, one step
at a time.

The next eleven days brought the challenges of eating, talking, thinking, dressing, standing, bathing, walking, going to the bathroom, most anything involving strength, endurance, balance, or coordination. My muscles had atrophied, and accomplishing these goals with diminished muscular strength felt like I was moving an inch at a time across a football field. At this point, I had no idea what level of independence I could accomplish. Sepsis had dealt me a stunning blow that shook me to the foundation of my being. I was still very deconditioned, tired, and lacked attention span, cognitive clarity, and overall motivation. It took a while to remember who I was before all of this happened. I needed to assess my situation realistically before I attempted to regain my overall physical and mental identity. Generating motivation would become a challenge on its own. I was an exhausted, atrophied mess wavering between just lying there and giving up, or changing gears and pushing it hard to regain my freedom, although placing one of those delicious chocolate milk shakes just out of reach might have inspired me to get out of bed.

I may not remember every doctor and nurse while I was caught in the crossfire of fever, infection, sepsis, and medications in the ICU, but here in the rehab hospital Dr. Patrick O'Brien, the medical director, was truly motivating and made quite an impression on me. He always took time to talk to me, and smiled throughout his visit, making me glad he stopped by. I called him the early morning cheerleader of hope. If he was around, the spirit was positive and uplifting. On follow up visits he always found something good to say about my progress like:"You're starting to get up on your walker, that's great."

In my room, I felt alone. It was the kind of loneliness that taunts you with despair while you are encapsulated in pain and suffering. I said to myself, "It's the bottom of a well I'm in, and I must look up and find my way out of here." I would not watch television. It was an aggravating buzz box of information that I didn't want to hear or process. I focused within, meditated, and prayed. I wanted hope to replace doubt, and faith to stifle my fear. I contemplated upon getting better. I wanted to turn off the other TVs. My roommate played his TV hour after hour until one or two in the morning, until I wanted to pull the wires out of the wall. The lady across the hall played hers so loud that I could hear it word for word at over twenty feet away. Sometimes a night nurse would be accommodating and ask them all to turn their TVs down or off. What a relief that was. I was isolated, but still content with the privacy curtain pulled three fourths of the way shut, with only a view of the door and hall remaining.

In the morning I could see a patch of uplifting blue sky just past the bricks around the window on my left, along with a small stream of sunlight as a silent friend. During the day there was new construction going on at a nearby building where another extension of the hospital was in progress. There were cranes creaking, and air hammers pounding old pavement into pieces. I heard the scraping sound of front end loaders scooping up dirt and debris, and rumbling exhaust pipes on heavy trucks as they pulled away in low gear. They strained from their heavy loads, as did I. This background construction symphony never bothered me. In fact, by Saturday morning I missed my Monday through Friday alarm clock that I had grown accustomed to.

My wife Nancy stocked the shelves in this room too. She provided a vast array of any food or drink item I requested, with a few creative inclusions of her own. There were containers of grape juice, apple juice, spring water, and Ensure nutrition shakes in several flavors. There were also multi-packs of mini cereal boxes, energy bars, peanut butter, blackberry jam, wheat bread and even fresh bananas. She also brought paper towels and napkins with cheerful designs on them. Every little bit helped my morale. She wanted me to get better, can't you tell?

While I struggled to recover in my prison of affliction, I continued listening to the construction symphony outdoors while the nurses zipped in and out to take care of me. Sometimes they checked my blood pressure or took blood samples, while other times it would be a routine shot in the stomach to help reduce blood clots. They also came in to patiently help me sit up and get out of bed, then on to a walker to go to the bathroom. Going to the bathroom was an exhausting process, fortunately insured by wearing adult disposable diapers, but nevertheless a daily challenge and accomplishment. It took all of my strength to pull and push until I could sit up. (This is where I may have overextended atrophied muscles causing nerve damage in my left shoulder that was discovered later).

The first few days a nurse would help me to sit up, until eventually I could get that far on my own. I still could not lift my legs off the bed to hang them down the side. They were still quite swollen and felt like heavy railroad ties. As the days progressed, I became able to get off the bed, stand precariously, and move a few feet with a walker. I could not stabilize enough to sit down in a chair, or get up from one. Again, I was exhausted. Every task seemed monumental to me. This included sipping from a straw, holding a cup, reaching for the nurse call button, and failing to unscrew caps from juice or spring water bottles.

During all of these frustrating situations, I was still wearing diapers and had a gallbladder tube coming out of my side and draining into a plastic bag attached to the bed rails. The bag filled with greenish brown bile that made you lose your appetite just looking at it. The tube and the drain bag went wherever I went, to the bathroom, strapped to a walker, or hung off the side of a wheelchair. I would have this attached to my body from July 24th until October 7th when I would have laparoscopic gallbladder surgery (cholecystectomy) and finally get rid of it. I really hated the painful tube coming out of my side. After I left the hospital I used a removable strap type drain bag attached with elastic below my knee. I drained it with a small valve on the bottom 3-4 times a day.

My first night in rehab, two female nurses bathed me in a heavy duty plastic chair. I didn't care if I was naked since I already felt completely stripped from my illness, and welcomed that first chair shower so much. It made me feel like I was making a new start, and washed away some of the torment and anguish of the previous weeks. It seemed to be liberating for my pent up emotional burdens too. All of this release and relief came in one shower. Afterwards, I struggled to stand up while they dried me off and dressed me in a clean hospital gown and a new diaper. I clambered onto a walker and slowly made it back to my bed with a nurse at my side.

The next morning, a nurse cheerfully came into my room with a wheelchair to take me to physical therapy. I did not want to get out of bed and do anything, but they had other plans. After 3-4 minutes of struggling to sit up, the nurse helped me slowly put on shorts, a t-shirt, socks, and shoes. I grabbed the edge of the bed and pushed myself into a wobbly standing position, then slowly took three steps to turn and drop into the wheelchair. The nurse held my gallbladder drain bag connected to the tube coming out of my side, and then strapped it securely to the underside of the chair so that it wouldn't tangle up in the spokes of the wheel. Then, one by one I lifted my legs up and set my feet on the fold down foot rests. This process took about ten minutes, and I was already tired from doing this. I now rolled along down the hall past a blur of rooms, people, and signs to the elevator. The bump at the door of the elevator felt like a pickup truck going over railroad tracks, then bump again when I got out. My body was very sensitive to any movement or vibration.

Soon I arrived at the physical therapy room. It was a huge L-shaped room full of mat tables, shelves with weights, parallel bars, training stairs, treadmills, exercise bikes, and other specialty equipment designed to restore strength and mobility. The atmosphere was quiet and focused for the most part, except for an occasional moan or groan from someone struggling to do their therapy, or gears and handles turning on some machine.

I quickly noticed that I was not the only person dealing with pain and suffering as I looked around the room. One elderly lady had a blue and purple face, and was straining to lift her arms up and down. A large, gentle looking man sat quietly with a protective helmet on his head. We smiled toward each other, peeking out from our painful existence to share a moment. Another older man looked extremely weary while he strained along with his male therapist who was helping him to sit up. He was supported with a chair propped behind his back. I felt the pain and dismay in his face. The therapist almost looked sad working with him, but kept a compassionate smile in place.

My physical and occupational therapists, Katey and Priti, were younger women with gentle smiles, kind spirits, and soft voices that guided me toward what seemed like impossible goals for my body. My exercises for strengthening and endurance for upper extremities included using dumbbells for bicep curls, chest presses, shoulder presses, lateral raises, and tricep extensions. Various leg lifts and bends were done for strengthening to regain balance and the ability to walk. My sessions began in a wheelchair, then after a few days I used a mat table, walker, and several exercise machines.

I came into this phase of my recovery in a weak, deconditioned state. I had lost weight and my muscles had atrophied. I was uncooperative and did not want to participate for the first two days. I was angry about all that had happened to me, and I sat sulking in my wheelchair. I felt like an old man with gray hair and a half-grown gray beard staring silently into a gray future. I didn't want anyone to place demands upon me to do anything. I just wanted to go back to my room, take pain medications and go back to bed. I didn't even want to eat.

Well, the therapists would not go along with my depressed avoidance and escapist disposition. They had other plans.

They were not going to let me drift off into self pity, so they encouraged me one step at a time toward my recovery, using a smooth combination of charm, motivation, and skill. This was the warm, compassionate health care that I needed, and received.

After a few days, God's love, peace, and power began to take over and lift me up. My energy had changed spiritually, mentally, and physically. My hope was no longer deferred, as faith and prayer gave me a positive visualization to go forward and overcome my obstacles. My therapists said that I picked up speed, increased my focus, and began to have remarkable gains in my rehab. There was a comeback in the making, and I could feel it in the air. I came out from behind my comfortable barriers and began to talk with my therapists and not just brush them off. I greeted the doctors and nurses with a more positive tone. I began talking to my roommate, and asked him how he was doing. I ate more of my meals too. I didn't just jump out of bed, or run down the hall on a walker, but I did make noticeable progress sitting up, eating, getting off and on my bed, and using the walker to go to the bathroom, as well as improvements in strength and endurance at my physical therapy sessions. But, most of all, there was a distinct change in my attitude which fed my desire to get better and leave the hospital.

As I felt a little stronger, I began to view my recovery like a confrontation or battle that needed to be won. "I must prevail against this enemy," I said to myself. I kept thinking about a scene in the 1982 movie First Blood, starring the amazing and intense Sylvester Stallone, who plays the hitchhiking veteran John Rambo returning home after serving in Vietnam. He is hassled by a local town sheriff (Brian Dennehy), thrown in jail, and abused and provoked until he overtakes the officers in an explosive escape up into the nearby mountains. In the ensuing chase by the sheriff and several other officers into the thick woods, Rambo's special military training kicks in and he takes the upper hand against his adversaries, and one by one begins to disable them. There is one particular scene where he ambushes the sheriff and holds him at knife point, demanding him to call off the pursuit. He says: "I could have killed them all; I could have killed you! In town you're the law, out here it's me. Don't push it! Don't push it or I'll give you a war you won't believe! Let it go! Let it go!"(Kotcheff, 1982).

Somehow, I harnessed Stallone's intensity, and became more aggressive, and faced off with my fears, pain and weakness. When I worked with Katey, one of my physical therapists, I would respond to her exercise requests with, "I'll give you a war you won't believe." It was not a war with her of course, but a war with my debilitated situation. I wanted to overcome it, so I worked as hard as possible each day.

I began doing more exercises. I bounced a huge exercise ball back and forth with one of the male assistants, and increased the distance I traveled on my walker. I also used a stepping machine, which was very difficult, and a rotating cycle exerciser with increasing resistance. This was done by grabbing handles and rotating in a bicycle motion. The therapist slowly increased the amount of repetitions and level of resistance to build me up. This was very tiring, but I kept at it with growing determination.

When I came back to my room after my daily sessions with the therapists, I was worn out. I took my pain medications and fell asleep before supper, and would have missed eating several meals if it were not for my wife and son waking me and helping me eat. They came to see me every day after work and made sure of it. I was very blessed to have wonderful and dedicated family support. This is very special to me and brings tears to my eyes. I noticed that some patients had only one visitor once in a while, and ate most of their meals alone while they watched TV. I was privileged and loved.

My days varied with activities other than physical therapy. They included tests and evaluations done by a speech pathologist, neuropsychologist, and ultrasound technician. Marcie, my speech pathologist, was very pleasant and patient while she tested my memory and cognition, and expressive and receptive language. She said I did well, but I did get a little sarcastic when I started drawing faces on the blank clock pages used for telling time. I guess I thought they were too easy and added some spice to it.

Another day, I visited Dr. Karen Wilhelm, a neuropsychologist. She was reserved, pleasant, and had a good sense of humor while she did my cognitive evaluation and assessment. The tests revealed mild deficits with attention, cognitive speed, verbal memory and initiation, visual memory, and mild disinhibition. I was still spinning in the wake of my traumas in the ICU. My encephalopathy was slowly resolving, but she needed to push me a little for responses. Requests to do things made me grumpy and less cooperative, but she said it was not unusual right after an acute illness. She was exceptionally patient and helpful as I more or less redefined my surroundings in the aftermath of the ICU and the transition into the rehab hospital. I enjoyed my visits with her, and felt encouraged.

Two nurses showed up one day and dashed me off for a long ride in my bed down several halls to get Doppler ultrasounds done on my legs. They were checking for any blood clots (deep vein thrombosis). Fortunately, all my test results were fine. The lighting in the room was subdued, and felt eerie. It was cold and gray and made me shiver. It was a pain-free process while they performed this medical imaging, but especially interesting when the nurse let me watch the monitor, or hear the unforgettable tones the sound waves made through the speakers. It sounded like an underground pump built by aliens who were sucking all of the thick tapioca out of a pudding factory back to their spaceship. I am glad I did not tell anyone, or I would have found myself in another ward of the hospital.

Group therapy was also done in a large meeting room that had a section with a wood floor, carpeted areas, a wide screen TV, piano, computers, and tables and chairs. Several patients were brought in wheelchairs to do minimal exercises in unison, and then took turns lapping the room on a walker if they could. Group sessions gave me a reality check that pointed out that I wasn't in solitary confinement, and others were dealing with recovery just like I was. Some patients looked lively while others could barely move, but most were glad to see someone else outside of the confinement of their rooms.

I missed my afternoon sessions one day because my doctor came in and wanted to run a test on my gallbladder performance. He turned off the drain valve on the tube coming out of my side to see how I would do without it. Within one hour I was in excruciating pain and the valve had to be reopened. When they came with a wheelchair to take me to physical rehab, I refused to go and could barely move in my bed. The nurse thought I was just being stubborn and contentious, but was not aware of the previous gallbladder test. It was explained to her the next day. I just stayed in bed until supper, still wondering how the gallbladder problem was going to be resolved.

After about nine days in rehab, a periodic reassessment was done at a team conference to discuss and document my progress, and to determine my discharge date from the hospital. Categories that were assessed included, medical, communication/cognition, mobility, and self care. I was eating 75-100% of all my meals, and was 100% continent with bladder and bowel control (which took a lot of patience and practice). My comprehension and expression were within functional limits, and my cognition had mild memory deficits, mild distractibility, and loss of focus. My bed mobility was independent, moving from a laying down position to sitting at the edge of the bed, or the reverse. Transferring from a bed to a chair or wheelchair, getting on and off the toilet, and getting up and down in a shower chair still required standby assistance with a helper nearby. I could do it, but it was very difficult. My walking distance with a rolling walker had increased to 150 feet, and I could travel 100 feet in a wheelchair on my own. I was reasonably independent with feeding and grooming tasks, but I needed a little help with upper and lower body dressing. My discharge would come in two days, but I didn't know it yet.

I could now eat my lunch sitting in a wheelchair, and afterwards wheel myself out of the room and down the hall about 40 feet, where I enjoyed looking out a window at trees bending in the wind and a sky full of puffy cumulus clouds. This was a very big step toward freedom. After lunch time, I was taken to a unique "practice apartment" in the occupational therapy department. They have a kitchen, living area, bedroom, and bathroom where you can work with a therapist to simulate at-home activities, such as getting on and off a bed or couch, or using the bathroom. The bedroom felt real with blankets and pillows on a queen bed, a dresser, and end tables and lamps, pretty much like home. I was taken here to test my skills for reentry into life at home. I got in and out of bed from my walker, got up and down in a chair, opened and shut full size curtains, and navigated to the bathroom and back. In the huge bathroom they have several different types of shower chairs available to try so that you can determine which one is best for your needs. My wife had provided us with the height, width, and depth of our bathtub to make sure the chair would fit. I selected a very nice wide, heavy duty 300 pound rated chair to purchase and take home. After selecting the shower chair, the medical equipment company that works with the rehab hospital delivers it to your room before you are discharged. They have excellent service, and make it convenient for you as a patient.

Adjacent to the WakeMed Rehab Hospital is the Health Park, which is specially designed to be a relearning indoor environment for patients. It has curbs, bridges, steps, various walking surfaces, plants, trees and park benches. There is also a putting green, fish pond, boat, full-size car and a walking track. The atmosphere is much like any other park, and provides a unique addition to health care. My wife brought me here in a wheelchair to enjoy a family visit in this beautiful setting, but I still was unable to climb steps, walk across bridges, or get in and out of a car.

WakeMed Rehab is an amazing place with a wide range of rehabilitation services that include medical care, inpatient rehab, day treatment, outpatient rehab, and home care. This patient-centered curriculum is implemented in a warm and compassionate atmosphere by doctors, nurses, and staff that care about their patients as much as they care for them. The WakeMed rehab team approach to my care, and treatment plan for recovery was successful. I greatly appreciate their commitment to me. My journey toward maximum rehabilitation and independence was well on its way.

On the 11th day, just after breakfast, a nurse came in and said the words I had been longing to hear, "You're going home today Mr. Black". Excitement filled the air as the nurses helped to prepare me to leave. The first nurse came in and reconnected my gallbladder tube (called a T-tube) to a different type of drain bag that would strap on to my lower leg with elastic bands. It had a valve at the bottom used to drain the bile for measuring and disposal. The tube coming out of my side was held by a stitch in the skin and covered with a gauze bandage for protection. I had to be very careful with it, and the bandage had to be changed every day.

I was given discharge instructions for follow-up appointments with a list of specialty doctors as needed, prescriptions for augmentin, oxycodone, and prilosec, and an appointment to return to rehab in about a month for evaluation of my progress. My wife and son arrived and helped a nurse's assistant pack up my clothes, personal items, containers, tape and bandages, back-up bile drain bag and tube, and huge shower seat. They stacked it all onto a cart. They threw away all of the food and drink items from the shelves just to be safe.

I gave a couple of nurses a hug and thanked them before we began our departure down the hall toward the exit, where my wife and son were waiting to take me home. It was a warm sunny morning full of optimism as we drove away from the hospital.

31 days had passed since my reeling entrance into the emergency room, my passage near death through the ICU, and my extended recovery in the rehab hospital. "Was I there that long?" I said to myself. My grasp of time continued to elude me as I embraced my day of discharge. My confinement came to a close. The war with sepsis had ended, and I was going home to face off with the aftermath.

CHAPTER SIX

THE RETURN HOME

Although the world is full of suffering, it is full also of the overcoming of it - Helen Keller

When I first came home, I was pleasantly surprised to see how Nancy had cleaned and rearranged the living room to give me space to use my walker. This is no easy task because our two-bedroom apartment is overflowing with stuff in every room, closet and hallway. My art work takes up about half of the kitchen and a third of the living room. She cleaned all of the carpets, washed the bedding and clothes, gave the bathroom a thorough scrub down, and stocked the refrigerator and cupboards with a wide variety of food and drinks. Whatever I needed, she took care of in a kind, patient and loving way. Her support was commendable and stellar to say the least.

I was happy to be home and eager to renew my life that had been suspended in a prison of affliction. But, I was very tired, touchy, and impatient and wanted quiet and uninter-rupted rest (which you do not get in the hospital). I slept a lot for the first four days, usually only 2-3 hours at a time, then the pain pills would wear off. My pain was extensive, and seemed to be everywhere at once. My body hurt as if my skin was a balloon with too much air in it, and my bones and muscles throbbed. I was constantly cold and shivering. The oxycodone barely helped me sleep. Once you hit a certain level of pain, not much helps. I still had the gallbladder tube in my side and the drain bag hooked up to it. It made it difficult to sleep in a regular bed because I worried about turning over and breaking the bag or tearing out the tube. It was also difficult to get in and out of bed with it in the middle of the night.

So, I slept in my recliner from August 20th to October 6th. It was just safer and more convenient for me, and gave my wife some needed uninterrupted sleep. She stayed home with me for the first four days and returned to work on the fifth day. The fifth day was the toughest for me because I was on my own to eat, drink, and use the bathroom unassisted. This period proved to be quite a struggle at times.

Nancy pampered me with my meals. When I got up out of the recliner in the morning, she had already left for work. My breakfast was cooked and waiting at the table, covered and still warm. A nice sandwich for lunch was already prepared and waiting in the refrigerator. I only needed to open it up and heat it in the microwave. I could not open jars, twist ties off of bread, take caps off of bottles, or handle any knives. I could barely get on my walker and make it into the kitchen or go to the bathroom. Afterwards, I took pain pills and went back to sleep for a while. Nancy also called me during breaks and lunch at work to check up on me and cheer me up. She is a remarkable woman, a dedicated wife, and best friend, with an overwhelming soulful personality full of kindness and love. I called her "super-woman" because she managed to do everything. She worked full time and extra hours, did all of the errands, cleaning, and meal preparations, washed dishes, did laundry, and waited on me anytime I needed something. She was simply amazing.

At the supper table, I would drift off easily, staring at my food, but not eating it, and missing parts of conversations. My wife and son kept an eye on me and urged me to eat when I did this. We celebrated getting out of the hospital one night by consuming a lot of expensive, sinfully delicious triple chocolate cake with layers of chocolate mousse in the center. It was so thick and rich that it dulled your senses by the time you finished, and no one even asked for a second piece. I had lost 25 pounds in the hospital, so I knew I could get away with this at least once.

After the first 4-5 days of resting and getting my home orientation into some focus, I began to deal with my new challenges. The aftermath of sepsis brought despair and hope, and I needed a bridge of faith to cross over to recovery. I could cave in, collapse, and give up, or choose to persist, endure, and eventually prevail. Staying positive was not always easy. Some days I sat there angry or depressed about my condition, while other days I pressed forward as hard as possible.

I needed to, and wanted to return to normal, physically, mentally, and spiritually. I had the challenges of: continuing my physical therapy for strength, balance, and coordination, regaining the ability to think clearly and focus, writing legibly, doing art work and playing guitar, and maintaining a positive visualization for success reinforced by faith, prayer, and divine intervention. The road to independence appeared winding and steep, and I had to travel it one difficult day at a time. The gallbladder tube remained in my side, and I had to carry the drain bag strapped to my leg through every daily activity. I had to drain it several times a day and measure the amount of bile and keep records for my surgeon, Dr. Rutherford. The gallbladder problem was unresolved and it worried me constantly.

It was heaven to be home, but it was hell to recover. I felt weak and small. My hell was my own, and I had to rise above it and refuse to be beaten. I was eclipsed by pain and suffering, yet there was light in my day, and there were stars in my dark nights. God gave me the strength to endure, and kept my inner flame burning.

My physical and occupational therapists sent me home with an extensive illustrated list of exercises to do for building strength and endurance. Some were done on my bed, in a chair, or while holding on precariously to my walker. The progress was slow and painful, and there were no charming therapists around to coach and encourage me. I missed them. My dumbbell exercises started out fairly well using 2-3 pound weights, but within one week diminished to a crawl because of my flared up shoulder injury. The damaged nerve caused excruciating pain, and my left shoulder drooped to the side. I couldn't reach or grab objects, and this just complicated my progress.

Doing leg exercises while holding onto the walker was difficult, because I had to strap the gallbladder drain bag to the metal frame and hold the drain tube out of the way while moving my legs up and down. If I made one mistake, I could tear the tube out of my side. I also had problems with the tube and bag when I showered. I strained to get off the walker and onto the shower chair, while I hooked the bag to a handle on the tub, and kept enough slack in the tube to move around while my wife helped me bathe. I got dizzy when I stood up to rinse off, and had to be very careful getting off the chair and stepping out of the tub to dry off, always watching the tube and drain bag so that nothing would get torn loose.

I practiced getting up and down out of a chair, and out of bed, but had to do that slowly too because the venous pooling in my legs made me very dizzy. This pooling was an accumulation of blood in the veins (of legs) due to gravitational pull when I changed positions from lying down to standing up. This took several weeks before it improved. I still had some edema in my ankles and feet which added pain and discomfort to standing. It slowly disappeared with the help of massages done by my wife, and my circulation improved. I built up the distance I could travel on my walker and felt less stress and more confidence with trips to the kitchen or the bathroom. Then I tested my walking with a cane, only a few feet at a time, but it was progress. After about two weeks I made it across the entire apartment. Getting braver, I tried walking without the cane. I looked a little inebriated while I grabbed chairs, tables, and door knobs to stabilize myself, but I kept going.

I went to my appointment with my surgeon, Dr. Rutherford on September 8th. He examined me and said that I wasn't strong enough for gallbladder surgery, and that I would have to walk into his office at my next appointment on the 23rd unassisted before he would consider doing the surgery. I accepted the challenge. The next day, September 9th, I got completely off my walker. I was a little wobbly, but remained determined to walk unassisted. As I began to accomplish some of my rehab goals, my layers of anxiety and fear began to peel off.

My handwriting was strained, shaky, and scribbled. I fought to regain control of my wrist and fingers, hoping to return to normal. I came up with the idea of using graph paper for physical therapy. I placed dots with a pen into the center of the squares, and then I drew diagonal lines across other squares for variations of focus and control. I did this over and over again, dots and diagonals, and I was successful with improving my coordination.

Drawing and guitar playing were my next challenges. "Can I do it?" I said hopefully. The first drawings were disappointing. I lacked concentration and control of pens and pencils, and it took several attempts before I felt comfortable sketching what I was seeing in my mind. I didn't quit, and over time I completed all of the illustrations in this book.

Guitar felt familiar, yet strange, because I could remember the chord shapes in my head, but my fingers were too weak and slow to form them on the fingerboard. I had the same problems playing scales. I would remember a major or minor scale, and then stumble through it. This was frustrating and discouraging because drawing, painting, playing guitar, and songwriting are my essential means of expression. I needed the mental acuity, hand-eye coordination, and strength in my fingers to combine smoothly to play like I used to. I had to be very careful, because holding the guitar would bump into the incision on my right side where the drain tube came out. I did not like that painful, cumbersome tube, but I knew it was helping me stay healthy. My guitar playing slowly reconnected. After about a month of uncomfortable and strained practicing, I began to play chords, chord progressions, scales, and arpeggios with much better control. It would take several months before I was back to my normal level of playing. I was very happy that I did not lose the ability to play guitar in the aftermath of my illness.

I wanted my life back. I wanted it the way it used to be, before sepsis turned everything upside down and inside out. I did not want to crawl along through each tiny increment of recovery, but I had to, there was no other choice. I felt like my life was buried under an avalanche of problems that would take forever to resolve. I sat in my recliner and sighed, then cried, while the air felt heavy to breathe. I felt the weight of my illness pressing in from all sides. Depression and sadness hovered over me like a dense fog making the future seem dim and hopeless.

The first 2-3 weeks were an emotional roller coaster. I had highs when I did something well and lows when it became too difficult. I needed to accept my limitations and confront the mounting turmoil within me. I got back on the right track through prayer, meditation, and visualization. I had to close out all of the negatives and distractions, and think peaceful, positive thoughts while I searched deep in my spirit. Then, I waited for a force greater than myself to lift me up to higher ground. I was open to it. God did this for me, and helped my physical, emotional, and spiritual gyroscope get back into balance. I needed that strength and stability to endure and overcome the days, weeks, and months ahead of me.

I had made it through the first three weeks and felt pretty good about going into the 4th week. I worked hard and poured out every ounce of determination into my rehab exercises, and increased the distance I could walk without a walker or a cane. I tired easily, and would nap for an hour after every workout. I read and wrote in my notebook to get myself focused mentally, and sketched some of my recollections of hospital episodes. Some of these memories were hard to deal with, but the art was therapeutic.

My rehab hospital follow-up appointment was September 18th. My wife took me because I was still unable to drive. Even though there were wavering moments, I walked from the parking lot into the hospital for my appointment. She carried a cane along, just in case I became too tired or weak. They tested my ability to walk, turn around, sit, and stand, then documented the complaint about my left shoulder and sent me for x-rays. They found some arthritis, but nothing damaged that might impair my shoulder mobility, so the pain continued without any resolution of the problem. They suggested using ice packs, but it didn't help at all. The walk to the x-ray lab was very long and tiring. I was offered a wheel-chair, but chose to rest a few minutes, and then walked back out of the hospital to the parking lot. My wife drove me home, and ten minutes after I got there, I fell asleep in the recliner.

The gallbladder was a nagging, painful problem and simply did not feel right. When I measured the bile in the drain bag, the daily total would vary from 40ml to 236ml per day. There was a constant deep, internal aching that made me very concerned. I discussed the gallbladder problem with Dr.

Rutherford and Dr. Whitt at my follow-up appointments on September 23rd.

My first appointment was with Dr. Rutherford. I walked into his office. He looked pleasantly surprised that I could do it, and shook my hand and congratulated me on my success. His challenge had been met! I was strong enough to walk into his office unassisted, which was his prerequisite for surgery. We discussed the pros and cons of the surgery to remove my gallbladder (laparoscopic cholecystectomy), and based on the intermittent performance of my gallbladder, and the constant pain, I elected to do it. The laparoscopic method would be the least invasive, with a shorter recovery period, but if he had any difficulty viewing the procedure, he said he would have to do open surgery with a large incision in my right side that would take a long time to heal. The gallbladder is not a vital organ, and fortunately you can live without it. He explained the procedure, the risks involved, and then scheduled me for outpatient day surgery in two weeks, on October 7th. We all felt comfortable with this decision.

Immediately after this appointment, I saw Dr. Whitt, my gastroenterologist. He told me that I was looking much better, back to a more normal appearance. We discussed the gallbladder surgery, and he agreed with the decision to remove it, and felt that I was now strong enough to endure it. Both doctors were optimistic about the upcoming surgery. My fears were quieted for the time being, as I cautiously looked forward to completing the surgery, and hopefully solving the gallbladder problem.

Dr. Rutherford went ahead and scheduled my pre-op appointment at the hospital for September 30th, which was seven days before my scheduled surgery on October 7th. I spent the next week doing my usual physical therapy, resting, eating balanced meals, and started taking all of my vitamins, minerals, and supplements from A to Z, with the exception of vitamin E which was discontinued because it could interfere with blood clotting. I waited through the days with mounting anticipation.

The pre-op appointment took a couple of hours. First, I went through registration. Then, I met with a nurse that documented my medical history, current medications, allergies, and diagnostic test results. They already had recent EKG's, MRI's, CT scans and X-rays, so I only needed to do blood and urine tests. I was also given detailed instructions to prepare me for surgery.

I met with an anesthesiologist to discuss my anesthesia care before, during, and after surgery. For me, pain control was a major concern. I was somewhat nervous about anesthesia, and not that trusting about the procedures because I had problems in past surgeries at other hospitals. When I had a phlebectomy (vein removal) done on my left leg, I woke up just before the doctor made an incision, and told him not to touch my leg. This set back the surgery for at least 15 minutes while they increased the amount of drugs and waited for me to pass out. Later in the recovery room, the nurse told me that they gave me enough to knock her out, and a couple of other nurses. Another time, I woke up in the operating room just after hernia surgery, while they were removing a large tube that went down my throat. I heard everyone talking and putting away surgical instruments and equipment, and felt excruciating pain in my groin, like a sword stabbing me. I even remembered the time on the round clock on the wall. There was no gradual return to consciousness, just shocking severe pain that made me tremble all over. I was crying out. My pain management was a disaster.

The WakeMed anesthesiologist listened to this history and responded with compassion, and reassured me that this would not happen with my gallbladder surgery. He discussed his credentials and experience working in both the ER and surgery departments, and I felt a lot better. Fortunately, no problems occurred with my surgery. The appointment and evaluation was over, and everything else was in place for my surgery. My return home became a progression toward a return to the hospital.

CHAPTER SEVEN

A LONGER ROAD

The greatest wealth is health - Virgil

It was October 7th, the day of surgery. I rocked back and forth on a seesaw of emotions. I was nervous, yet hopeful and relieved to finally confront my gallbladder problem. I struggled to overcome my anxiety. I was worried about the possibility of having open surgery with a large incision in my side, and a more painful, prolonged recovery time. If the surgeon encountered any difficulties using the minimally invasive laparoscopic procedure to remove my gallbladder, he would have to choose to do open surgery. Although open surgery occurs in only a small percentage of cases, it remained in the back of my mind.

I didn't eat or drink anything after midnight the night before, and I prayed and tried to quiet my apprehension so that I could get a good night's rest. I woke up before the alarm clock went off, had a quiet, comforting shower, and brushed my teeth and got dressed in loose, comfortable clothes and slip-on shoes. I put notes everywhere, on the refrigerator, my dresser, and on doors and cupboards, reminding me not to eat or drink anything. I read them several times as I paced back and forth waiting to leave for the hospital.

My WakeMed day surgery was scheduled for 1:00pm. I was required to be there two hours early by 11:00am, so my wife, son Dorian, and I left at about 10:30am. She drove me because I couldn't handle it yet. My mental acuity and physical coordination just weren't up to par for the responsibility of driving. We arrived on time at the Day Surgery Center and checked in at the information desk, where I was given a number that they called when Patient Registration was ready to register me. They called my number, then verified all of my information, and placed an identification band on my wrist. Now, I went to the Day Surgery Reception desk where I received a pager which was used as a communication tool while at the center, whenever it blinked and buzzed I had to go to the desk for further instructions.

My next stop would be pre-operation preparation in the Day Surgery Center, which would take about an hour. I was alone now, while my wife and son waited in the lobby and the nurses did the prep work. Pre-op preparation included verifying my patient identification and information, the kind of surgery I was having, and then removing my clothes, getting into a hospital gown and then into bed, and placed in a small room with one chair and heavy sliding curtains. Another nurse came in and attached heart monitors and inserted an IV into my arm. Once I was completely prepped and covered in blankets (the rooms are usually cold), my wife was allowed to visit me in the pre-op room. It was now 12:45pm, with only 15 dragging tense minutes to go. My wife and I prayed and waited. My surgeon, Dr. Rutherford, stopped by with a brief cheerful visit just to check on my condition and encourage me, then left to get ready in the surgery room.

It was 1:00pm. The curtains were drawn back and I heard someone say in a positive, energetic tone, "We're ready for you Mr. Black!" I barely got to say goodbye to my wife as the nurses whisked me out of the room, and rolled me down the hall to the operating room. The room felt cold and sterile, and the lighting was bright, but not warm and comforting. Everyone had masks on, but their eyes revealed warmth and concern. They spoke in a kind orderly manner and asked me my name, what kind of surgery I was having, and verified the correct location on my body where the surgery was to be performed.

They carefully transferred me to the operating table and double checked my monitors and IVs. I would only hear two more voices. I recognized them both. First, my anesthesiologist talked to me and reassured me that everything was under control as he started my anesthesia. Then, in a few brief words, and in his usual cheerful tone, Dr. Rutherford asked me how I was doing. I said fine, and then asked God to help the doctors and nurses with my surgery. That was all I could remember. There was no slow countdown or hazy retreat from consciousness, just "blink!" like a light switch and I was out.

My laparoscopic cholecystectomy (gallbladder removal) was successful, without complications. That was great news to wake up to in the recovery room. No large incision with open surgery was required. My fears subsided and I finally relaxed. Dr. Rutherford made a quick stop in the recovery room to let me know that everything went fine, and then zipped off to the next patient. He looks busy when he's standing still.

Gallbladder removal by laparoscopic surgery is a unique procedure that requires only four small openings in the abdomen. Four narrow tubes called laparoscopic ports are placed through the tiny incisions for the laparoscopic camera and instruments. A laparoscope (which is a long thin round instrument with a video lens at its tip) is inserted through the belly button port and connected to a special camera which provides the surgeon with a magnified view of the internal organs on a television screen. The abdomen is inflated with harmless carbon dioxide gas for easier viewing, and to provide room for the surgery to be performed. Long specially designed instruments are inserted through the other three ports for removal of the gallbladder. The gallbladder is delicately separated from its attachments to the liver and the bile duct, and is removed through one of the ports. After the removal, the small incisions are closed with only a few small stitches below the belly button, and Dermabond topical skin adhesive is brushed over the wounds. This adhesive provides a microbial shield while working as a bonding agent that holds the incisions together. It wears off naturally during the healing process. This type of minimally invasive surgery offers several benefits such as: less post operative discomfort since incisions are smaller, quicker recovery time, a shorter hospital stay, and an earlier return to normal activities.

I was ready to go home by 5:00pm, but had to wait a while for a resident doctor to change an incorrect prescription so that I would go home with the correct pain medications. While I waited in the wheelchair, my pain slowly escalated and I began to feel the incisions in my abdomen, and soreness in my chest and sides. I was so glad to get rid of the gallbladder tube and drain bag, and have a successful laparoscopic procedure, rather than having a large incision in my side, that I continued to maintain a cheerful spirit.

I was soon released from the hospital and wheeled down the hall with my son by my side, and then out the door to our mini-van where my wife was waiting. I carefully eased into the seat and held a pillow over my abdomen while the seat belt was hooked up for me. It took a couple of minutes to get settled. I noticed every bump and turn in the road on the way home, even though my wife drove very carefully. It was a huge relief to get back.

The arduous task of recovery became two steps forward and one step back. The seismic shock of sepsis had somewhat subsided, but the gallbladder surgery left me in a fragile state. My steps forward were slow and painful. I already had two incisions from the gallbladder tube installation and reinstallation. Four more incisions were added from the surgery bringing it to a total of six incisions that gave me a very touchy side and stomach area. My physical therapy came to a halt, while I readjusted to quite a lot of pain, more than I expected actually. I took oxycodone for pain every 4 hours, and slept a lot for the first three days.

I was back in my normal bed at last! The burdensome gallbladder tube and drain bag were gone, but it was still difficult getting up and down out of bed because it tugged on my surgical incisions. It was equally difficult using the bathroom or getting in and out of a chair. Although I went home the same day of the surgery, I did not return to normal activities within a week's time. My recovery was progressive, but slow and painful. The months of rehab from the aftermath of severe sepsis had simply worn me out, and I had just begun to walk unassisted and complete my daily exercises. I rested, and then reassessed my situation. I began pacing myself as I worked toward my goals and objectives, which included driving a car and managing daily needs smoothly and independently. Reconditioning took about three weeks, and the healing process trudged onward at a snail's pace. My pain would come and go, and sometimes it became cumulative, and hit me really hard to the point where I was shaking and felt like crying. My upper back and left shoulder had extreme pain with a limited range of motion in my entire left arm. This problem continued to nag me and limit my recovery, so I had to just take it easy.

My other son Adrian and his wife Kari came to visit for a week. They were there for me for several days back in the ICU at the hospital, and after I returned home, and it was very supportive and encouraging that they came again. I felt more alive and energetic with my family around me, and it helped take the focus off of my pain and suffering. Love and care are great medicines for the mind, body, and spirit.

My hair started to fall out a few days after surgery, leaving a little here and there on a towel or a hair brush. Within two weeks, I lost 30-40% of it, and it only added to my frustrations. I wondered if it would grow back, or if I would need to start buying a lot of cool hats. I said to myself, maybe I should grow back the coarse gray beard I had at the Rehab Hospital. The nurses and therapists seemed to like it. My few moments of vanity and concern for self-appearance vanished quickly as I grappled toward normalcy like someone crawling upward out of a well, clutching one crevice at a time.

I felt a lot of internal turbulence throughout October. Summer was gone and fall was approaching, and my recovery felt uneasy. Sometimes I felt like my colors had run dry, and I was a tree losing its leaves to an overpowering stormy wind. Other days felt full of promise and hope as if complete success was just around the corner if I could hold on a little longer. Some days were more bearable than others, but I went forward as God helped me to slowly get back in tune with myself.

November was full of activity. I had several follow-up appointments to go to, and tests to try to determine what was wrong with my painful shoulder. On November 4th, I saw Dr. Rutherford, my gallbladder surgeon. I weighed in at 211 pounds, which was a 25 pound weight loss from the 236 I weighed when I first went into the hospital. He said that I looked great, and that it would take 2-3 more months for my metabolism to return to normal, with weight possibly returning, so watch the calories. He asked me, "Do you miss your little friend?" referring to that awkward and painful gallbladder tube and drain bag. "Yeah sure," I replied as he radiated a big smile. He is a great doctor and a pleasant guy with a good sense of humor. One of his nurses said that he has "a twinkle in his eye." I showed him some of my first sketches. He liked them and asked to make copies right there in the office, and also requested an autographed copy of my book, whenever I got it published. He recommended visiting everyone in the ICU, and contacting the Public Relations office of WakeMed to obtain consent to do interviews and gather information for this book. He pointed out that some people in the ICU don't remember a thing, while others have a clear memory of events. I remembered a good portion of some events, and pieces and parts of others. The research and interviews helped put the puzzle together. We discussed the chronic shoulder problem and he gave me a referral to an orthopedic doctor for further examination of the dysfunction, atrophy, and weakness.

My wife and I were at the hospital from 9:30am until 3:00pm that day. One appointment was in the morning, and afterwards we ate lunch in the cafeteria. I popped into the physical therapy room and said hello to a couple of therapists, and thanked them again for their kindness and patience with my recovery, and even got a hug from one of the ladies. We then went to the afternoon rehab appointment, where they tested my walking skills and discussed my shoulder problem. They agreed with Dr. Rutherford's referral to orthopedics and sent me on my way. We got home about 4:00pm and I faded to sleep very quickly in my recliner. I was in slow motion the next morning. I really felt the physical impact from walking all over the hospital, but I also felt very happy about being able to do it, even if I was under a certain amount of strain. I got back into the rhythm of my exercises over the next few days, and started to do laps walking around our apartment building too.

On November 11th, I went to see Dr. Mark L. Wood at Wake Orthopedics, as a referral from Dr. Rutherford. He gave me a thorough and patient examination and found significant ptosis (drooping) of the left shoulder with prominent winging of the scapula, and atrophy around the shoulder girdle. The winged scapula was evident in both the "wall-push test", and in the three x-rays of the left shoulder. This is a condition where the scapula is abnormally positioned outward and backward, giving a wing-like appearance where the shoulder blade on the upper back protrudes backward rather than lying mostly flat. Damage or impingement of a nerve can result in weakening or paralysis of the muscles, causing pain and limited shoulder elevation. Dr. Wood felt that my left shoulder dysfunction most likely represented a neurapraxia (nerve damage) of some sort, possibly caused by a traction injury in the ICU. Neurapraxia refers to temporary failure of nerve conduction due to blunt injury or compression, which can bruise or stretch a nerve. My symptoms included numbness, tingling, burning pain and muscle weakness. In order to rule out other causes of my dysfunction, and atrophy and weakness, he recommended an MRI of my cervical spine, brachial plexus, and left shoulder, and EMG nerve conduction tests.

Meanwhile, I continued painfully doing my range of motion and strengthening exercises. The healing progress was very slow, with occasional moments of freedom from pain. The range of motion in my shoulder appeared to be increasing as I worked out with dumbbells, but the pain and weakness persisted. Sometimes I would feel stronger and help with light chores, but I got tired very quickly. By November 18th I noticed that my hair was starting to grow back, just a little at a time, but it was great news! Dr. Rutherford had told me it would grow back. I guess the hat collection would have to be put on hold. Two days later on November 20th I finally drove my mini-van! I had not driven a vehicle for 4 months, so this was an exciting event that lifted my spirits. I only drove to the grocery store and back, but I felt like all of the physical therapy finally gave me a sense of independence.

On November 25th, the day before Thanksgiving, I went back to WakeMed hospital for my MRIs. My overall condition continued to improve, but I was not confident enough to drive in heavy traffic or on the freeway, so my wife drove me. I was hoping that these tests would finally reveal just exactly what was wrong with my shoulder. I was placed in a traditional MRI unit that is a large cylinder-shaped tube surrounded by a circular magnet. I was given a panic button placed next to my hand in case of any emergency. I lied on my back strapped onto a movable examination table, which slides into the center of the magnet. I opted for headphones with classical music to help me relax and block out the noises of the MRI scanner, but it wasn't that successful. The machine drowned out the music quite often and was frustrating. The magnetic field and pulses of radio energy used to produce the imaging created loud tapping, thumping, buzzing, and humming noises that are distinctive sounds found only in an MRI machine. Combine the sounds of a washing machine spinning way out of balance with warning buzzers going off at a nuclear plant, and stray radio signals from Mars and you would be close.

If you have claustrophobia, anxiety, or difficulty remaining perfectly still, you will not be happy in the MRI cylinder. The space is very confined, and some people require sedation to manage. I spent a total of 90 minutes in the MRI machine with only two one-minute breaks to readjust and reposition straps and bracing devices. That is a long time to lie perfectly still without becoming startled or panic-stricken. I prayed, meditated, and breathed in and out slowly and centered on a quiet place in my mind and spirit which helped me achieve success. I lost track of time and before you know it the MRIs were completed, and I was congratulated by the technician for completing an MRI marathon. Now, I would have to wait for the results. Waiting was made easier because Thanksgiving was the next day, and I would enjoy a great meal with family around me, so I didn't think about it much. I was having great difficulty gaining any weight back. I could eat just about anything and not gain an ounce past 211 pounds. Apparently my metabolism had not returned to normal yet, and the healing process was consuming all of the calories. Yes, I had two pieces of pumpkin pie with whipped cream towering on top, and ice cream too! It was a carpe diem opportunity, so I took it. My weight remained at 211 pounds when I checked it after Thanksgiving, and stayed that way until Christmas.

I called back Dr. Wood's office on Monday, November 30th to inquire about the MRI results, and see if I would still need to do the EMG tests. I was hoping to escape them, but the MRIs were not conclusive so they scheduled me for EMG's on December 9th. The weeks went by. My shoulder injury continued to trouble me. My range of motion had increased allowing me to elevate my arms and reach for things, but I was still very limited in duration of activity. The pain just made everything freeze up.

On December 9th, I went to see Dr. Richard Tim at Raleigh Neurology Associates, where an EMG-nerve conduction study was performed. I had been trying to avoid these tests, and hoped that the x-rays and MRIs would identify the painful shoulder problem, but they weren't conclusive and really didn't show any definitive causes so I had to deal with the EMG tests.

There are two parts to the test, the nerve conduction study and the needle EMG study. First, I changed clothes and got into a hospital gown. Then, two technicians came in and attached electrodes on my shoulder, arm, and hand with a tape-like adhesive. During the first part, called the nerve conduction study, brief electrical impulses or shocks were sent along the course of my shoulder and arm causing a snapping sensation, feeling something like static shock when you touch a metal door handle after shuffling across a carpet. The impulses are read by electrodes attached to various points, and the intensity of the impulses is increased causing muscle contractions or twitching that was mildly uncomfortable. The amount of current is kept at a safe level. This test took 25-30 minutes because they stop to read the monitor and make calculations and chart the results of the nerve functions. It does become annoying as they increase current levels, because the snapping sensation gets worse and causes some discomfort. I needed to find out just what was wrong with my left shoulder and trapezius area, so I was willing to do whatever tests were needed.

The second part of the study is called the needle examination, which involves inserting very thin needles into your muscles, which are microscopic electrodes that pick up normal and abnormal electrical signals given off by the muscle. The EMG needles are used only on you, and are not recycled, and are immediately disposed of following use. The needle is inserted in the relaxed muscle and moved inside to record muscle activity which is amplified by the EMG machine. It makes a crackling sound similar to static or bad reception on a radio. This is the part of the test that I was anxious about, first because I have never had it done, and second because others have told me how bad it was.

Dr. Tim came in the room, greeted me briefly, and got right down to business. He had me lift up my hospital gown for access to my back, neck and shoulder, and then roll over on my side which was uncomfortable from gallbladder surgery scars. After he got me into the position he wanted, he told me he was going to do 6 insertions with the needles, and then began immediately, not giving me any time to think about it. When the needle is inserted, it is painful and uncomfortable and the muscle feels cramped, but it is a tolerable procedure, especially if you relax and focus on something else. I kept thinking that this was nothing compared to the pain I endured in the ICU, and I did not moan or say a word once during the procedure. In this test, the needle probe is a recording device and no electrical shocks are given. The test lasted about 20 minutes, with the final insertion done at the bottom of my neck near my shoulder. This one was the most painful, and I was relieved that he was finally finished.

This needle insertion was bleeding, and the doctor had to put some gauze on it until it stopped. There was also a bloody spot on the pillow about the size of a quarter. Dr. Tim told me to get dressed and then left the room for about ten minutes. When he returned he told me the short version of the results. I had a damaged nerve, but it was growing back, and it would take a long time. He did not estimate how long it would take, and only indicated that he expected clinical improvement to occur.

His summary and interpretation in my EMG-nerve conduction study records indicated that the study was abnormal, with evidence of a left spinal accessory mononeuropathy. The EMG of the left arm and shoulder was notable for denervation and reinnervation changes in the trapezius, with ongoing reinnervation in the trapezius.

Somewhere in the hospital process (possibly pulling myself up in my bed, or from being moved in the ICU or for tests) I injured my shoulder which resulted in mononeuropathy (damage to a single nerve or nerve group) which caused denervation (loss of nerve supply), constant pain, and limited use of my arm and shoulder. Reinnervation, (restoration of nerve function) was going to take a long time. There would be no easy fix here, and I would have to tough it out with physical therapy and some massages. When I got home after the tests, I had to put an ice pack on my upper back where the bleeding insertion was done. It felt better in a couple of hours, but was noticeable for a couple of days.

Two days later, on December 11th, I returned for my follow-up appointment with Dr. Wood. He came in the door smiling and told me the good news, that I would not need surgery, and that the x-rays and MRIs did not reveal any structural damage. He told me about the damaged nerve, and the indications that the nerve was growing back, and recommended that I continue my range of motion exercises. So, it was pretty much up to me now. I had to be diligent with exercise to improve atrophied muscles, and patient with the reinnervation process of my left spinal accessory nerve. Sometimes my shoulder felt compressed and tight, and the nerve pinched. My shoulder drooped at times, and pulling, pushing, and extending my arm would be painful and sluggish.

It took several months for the pain and pinching in my shoulder to diminish and become manageable, and for my strength to increase so that I could accomplish daily tasks. It has not gone away completely, and I am writing this page 11 months later. If I use the shoulder conservatively it is tolerable and I can perform most activities such as doing laundry, driving, or playing guitar. I can't do repeated lifting such as carrying in groceries, or sitting in one position writing or working at the computer for more than an hour or two. I still work out with dumbbells and my wife and son massage my shoulder and back. Massage therapy can get pretty expensive.

It was December 16th, and in my notes I wrote:"I'm a walking, talking miracle," as I pondered enduring and surviving severe sepsis, having successful gallbladder surgery, and recovering slowly from nerve damage in my shoulder. I was not completely, 100% back to normal, but I was managing quite a bit at 80-90% recovery. I went ahead and gathered my ideas together for the content of my book, researched about sepsis and stayed up late at night drawing my experiences in small sketch books. I spent hours and hours collecting information and getting in tune with myself, so that I could capture the mental and spiritual aspects of my battle with sepsis in my writing and my art work. This process was tiring and draining, but also revealing and even liberating at times.

I took a week off from writing and doing research. I needed to relax and do nothing. It was time to get away from thinking about sepsis, hospitals, tests, doctors, and suffering. 2009 was coming to a close as I enjoyed a peaceful, quiet Christmas. I was blessed to be able to continue participating in life, to laugh, to love, to cry, and to triumph in the human spirit and beyond. The gifts of life and love from my wife and family made it a wonderful, joyful Christmas.

January and February of 2010 were full of inspiration and hard work on my book. My recovery had peaked at 85-90%, and I struggled with my shoulder injury and regaining my energy and endurance. I worked day and night and even in my sleep, sometimes jumping out of bed at 3:30am to jot something down. I ate balanced meals and extra protein bars, slept six hours at night with a one-hour afternoon nap, and continued all of my physical therapy. I worked on the internet, visited libraries and bookstores, and made phone calls to try to arrange interviews with my doctors. I developed an interview form to use at the hospital and with family members, to gain more knowledge and insight about my entire hospital experience. My surgeon, Dr. Rutherford suggested contacting the WakeMed Public Relations office to obtain consent to interview and gather information, so on January 13th I met with Heather Monackey who gave me an official signed consent form, and also assisted in setting up meetings with WakeMed Hospital staff members. I completed Dr. Rutherford's interview by phone, and meanwhile I gave all of my family members an interview form to complete.

On January 20th I returned to Dr. Whitt's office for a follow-up visit and an interview for my book. He told me that I was looking good and gave me a lot of time for an interview. We discussed my physical condition, disposition, and behavior when he initially met me about the 7th day in the ICU, and the care he gave me. He described my condition as acutely ill, with evolving multi-organ failure (a result of sepsis), and paranoid and scared. He ordered ultrasounds, a liver biopsy, ruled out Wilson's disease and prescribed mucomyst for acetaminophen toxicity. He felt that my baseline mental and physical health and my family support were keys to my survival. Coming into the hospital in good shape was an advantage. When I was in the ICU for 14 days, I was very skeptical of doctors and did not trust anyone. Dr. Whitt approached me quietly and patiently, and took time to talk with me in a calm pleasant manner, and I reacted to him as a more cooperative, trusting patient. Dr. Whitt even sent me a second interview response where he reiterated and elaborated about my case. He is an excellent doctor who is pensive and inquisitive, with gears always turning as he searches diligently for answers. He liked my art work and encouraged me to work on this book, and even copied an article about sepsis for me to help out.

After I left his office, I went to the bottom floor of the hospital to the records office. I waited about 25 minutes for all of the copies to come through the system, and left with about 100 pages of hospital records that detailed all 31 days of my stay from the time I entered the emergency room up to the day I was discharged from the Rehab Hospital. These records proved to be very helpful in writing this book. I took the records home and slowly read them page by page, which gave me a mounting realization that surviving sepsis was a blessing from God. This was not easy to do. Sometimes, I would stop reading and flash back to a trembling desperate moment in the ICU, or I would drift off through memories of rehab or find myself struggling on a walker to go to the bathroom. In the final analysis, reading it all made me more thankful to be alive, and more knowledgeable to accomplish writing this book.

My next interview was on February 5th with Dr. Micchia, my primary care physician. We did it at the end of the day at about 5:30pm after office hours. I enthusiastically thanked him again for his diagnostic accuracy about the sepsis, and his expedience in getting me to the emergency room back on July 20th, 2009. He appreciated my gratitude and said:"It makes my day to hear that!" He told me I was very lucky to have survived my ordeal with severe sepsis, and that he had been worried about me. We had a good discussion about my progress, and I showed him several of my drawings that expressed my ordeals in the ICU. He responded by saying: "Is there any Heaven at the other end?" I told him that I learned several positive life changing lessons from the hell I had been through, and that I would write about it in my book. I am so glad that I got to talk with him. He also re-quested a signed copy of my book.

On February 10th I called Dr. Rutherford at home. He agreed to do a phone interview because he has an extremely busy and constantly changing schedule, as well as crowded office hours. He described my condition back in the ICU as "sick." That sounded simplified, but he explained that when the term "sick" is used among surgeons it means that your condition is very bad, and in my case, too sick for any operation. He felt that the sepsis was not caused by my gallbladder, and that something else made the gallbladder sick. They found nothing in my cultures. The source of the sepsis was un-known, and has remained that way. That is a scary fact. He decided to have the gallbladder tube installed on the 4th day in the ICU, and saw me every day while he hoped and waited for my recovery. I didn't leave the hospital until August 20th, and had surgery much later on October 7th. I thanked him again for taking good care of me, and for being another one of the warm, compassionate health care professionals at WakeMed Hospital. "How did I get so many great people?" I asked him. He replied, "Somebody up there was looking out for you!" ♡

In between interviews, phone calls, and research on the internet and library, I constructed a timeline that went from July 2009 to July 2010, and also an outline of chapters for my book. I drew the timeline and the chapter outline on 22"x28" poster board, and posted them on the bedroom and bathroom doors where I could easily see them at a glance while I was working. This really helped me unify my thoughts and reconstruct all of the events that had transpired.

February 23rd, 2010 was interview day at WakeMed Hospital, set up by Heather Monackey at WakeMed Public Relations. It's not that easy to contact busy hospital staff members, and line up a meeting that fits their schedules. After waiting several weeks, a meeting was scheduled for me at the Health Park classroom, where I had the opportunity to interview my two therapists Katey and Priti, speech pathologist Marcie, and clinical neuropsychologist Dr. Karen Wilhelm. Although we were squeezed for time during their lunch hour, it went well, and I appreciated them taking the time for me. After everyone arrived in the classroom, I took a few moments to describe my book and why I was writing it. Then, I showed them the cover design and several sketch books with drawings depicting various episodes and events that transpired in the hospital. We had a combination of group discussion and individual interviews, and the atmosphere was cheerful and positive.

The basic format for discussion included describing my physical condition, my disposition and behavior, the type of care they gave me, and any significant situations or events that occurred while I was their patient. Overall, I was described as a good patient, but I was weak, deconditioned, and not always cooperative when asked to perform particular tasks. Katey and Priti both said that after a few slow, struggling days I picked up speed and had remarkable gains in my rehab, and Marcie said I did well on my memory and cognition tests. Dr. Wilhelm said that I did everything that I was asked to do in my cognitive screening, and that I had some mild difficulties with short term memory and speed on thinking. I know that I was grumpy and sometimes uncooperative with her, but she was very patient, understanding, and compassionate while working with me. She explained that it was not unusual to be less cooperative right after an acute illness. I think that my pain and suffering caused me to be withdrawn and depressed at times, and then I would just shut everyone out and hide inside. All of these wonderful and professional staff members helped me to overcome these obstacles.

Time ran out quickly for my brief reunion with these great WakeMed staff members that helped pull me through my recovery. They did a fantastic job, and I thanked them again for being warm, compassionate, and professional with my care. Dr. Wilhelm reminded me to also be sure to give myself some credit for overcoming my obstacles. I can only respond by thanking God for the strength to do it. We had a great meeting, and it was wonderful to see everyone again.

Immediately after the classroom interviews, I went to my 1:00pm appointment with Elaine Rohlik, executive director of Wake Med Rehab Administration. I received a warm welcome in her office. I briefly described my harrowing encounter with severe sepsis, and the blessed, remarkable recovery I had in their hospital. I told her that WakeMed gave me a warm, compassionate, and professional atmosphere unlike any hospital I have ever encountered. I called it the healing power of compassionate health care, a positive vibe that was very important to my recovery. Elaine responded by pointing out that WakeMed Rehab is a patient-centered curriculum where the staff is expected to "care about" their patients as much as they "care for" them. Administration reinforces this curriculum, and considers compassionate, patient-centered care a prerequisite for employment on the staff. We discussed the basic outline of my book, and I showed her the cover design and several pages of art work. I think she liked the art work, but as many people do, she made some perplexed facial expressions while viewing some of the dream and delirium sketches. She was very encouraging about doing the book, and hoped it would make a positive impact for others. It was a real pleasure to do her interview. Elaine is really charming, and a radiant ambassador for the hospital. She even sent me a thank you card afterwards.

After her appointment, I went to the hospital cafeteria for lunch. I had been talking with five different staff members for over two hours, and I was tired, but I felt like I had accomplished a lot, gaining more insight into everything that transpired. I had a sandwich and some coffee and rested for a while, before I took the long walk back through the hospital to the parking lot. I left at 11:00am and returned at about 3:30pm that day, and when I got home I headed for my recliner and fell asleep until supper.

The momentum of my book continued to grow as I collected information from interviews, books and articles, and a video on sepsis, which I compiled into folders. There were several folders with research about sepsis, and others with information about book layouts, famous quotes, near-death experience, and hospital procedures. Page after page, my work piled up until the folders were bulging with several hundred pages of information.

February went by quickly, and I had three more phone interviews to complete in March. Two would be with my male nurses in the ICU, and the third with my internal hospitalist on the 6th floor. Back in the ICU, I was cared for by several doctors and nurses on different shifts. I don't remember them all, in fact only a few like Dr. Whitt and Dr. Rutherford, and vaguely Mike and Drew, the two registered nurses who spent a lot of time with me.

Mike told me that he has seen a lot of sepsis cases, and that I was heading downhill and my mental status was deteriorating. I was paranoid and it was hard to tell if I was joking, serious, or out of my head at times. He noted that I had excellent family support, and that my sons, Dorian and Adrian were willing to assist him at anytime they were needed, such as lifting and moving me or talking with me when I was upset. He described some of the equipment used on me in the ICU, and explained why the PICC line was moved to my neck after I ripped it out. I thanked him for taking time to talk with me in a reassuring way in the ICU, and that his compassionate and professional care made a difference.

Drew said that I came into the ICU very sick, and then got worse. I had high temperatures and became very swollen and completely yellow. He said that I was talkative, but confused and told him interesting stories. He described most of the equipment that he used on me, and said that sepsis is common in the ICU, and that he sees it every week. I also thanked him for taking good care of me. Somehow, they both managed to ignore my paranoia and conspiracy stories and continued their daily care of me. I greatly appreciated their kindness and patience, especially since I wasn't always cooperative or aware of what was going on, and I had a tendency not to trust anyone that came in the room.

After 14 days in the ICU, I was taken to the 6th floor to begin my long road to recovery. Here, Dr. Alisha Benner, internal hospitalist, helped me to make my transition. A hospitalist is a physician whose primary professional focus is the general medical care of hospitalized patients. She called me at home to do an interview. We spent nearly half an hour talking about the special help that I needed in my deconditioned physical state and my altered mental state. I was unable to do many activities and felt helpless and confused. Besides my maintenance care, she spent a lot of time talking to me and offered comforting words and positive support, especially when I would perseverate about dying or exhibit circular thinking. I closed the interview by thanking her for the gentle and kind care that she gave me.

I had several other staff members that I wanted to interview, but they were simply unavailable. The hospital is a very busy place. I still felt that I had enough information that I could continue writing my book. When you are in extreme pain and spinning in eddies of the aftermath of a severe illness, it is easy for names, faces, and moments of time to become distorted memories. So, the interview process proved to be a good idea, and by the end of March I had over a dozen folders filled with information.

While still struggling with a slowly healing, damaged nerve in my shoulder, I had two other problems that added mileage to my road of recovery. One was sexual performance, and the other was an itchy skin condition on two fingers of my left hand.

The most severe, unrelenting problem has been the itchy skin condition called scabies, which is caused by tiny mites that burrow under the skin, lay eggs and multiply. The symptoms include pimple-like irritations or a rash (which spreads quickly) and intense agitating itching. The itching is more intense at night or after a hot shower. It's worse than poison ivy and it is nearly impossible not to give in and scratch the infected area. I call them the itch mites from Hell that just won't die. It is acquired through close contact with an infected individual or contaminated clothing, towels, or bedding. It can spread quickly where there is frequent skin to skin contact between people, such as nursing homes, child-care centers or hospitals. I have no idea how I acquired the scabies. The condition did not appear until two months after I returned from the hospital. I went to my doctor and he prescribed Permethrin which is a scabicide. I also use a 10%

formula of sulfur soap to scrub my fingers. This condition has persisted for months while I have been writing this book. I wondered if my battle with severe sepsis left me with a weakened immune system, which is causing the skin condition to heal at a much slower pace. I wash all of my bedding, and scrub my fingers with soap and water several times a day. I put medications on at night, and if the itching starts driving me crazy I use calamine lotion too. Hopefully this horrible condition will be gone before I finish this book.

Recovering from sepsis had an impact on my sex life and sexual performance. This problem is not about senior sex or buying products to rekindle and relive youthful desire and stamina. This is about overcoming the aftermath of sepsis. I was left so physically beat up from massive scrotal swelling in the ICU, that I didn't even think about sex for months, and when I did, my self confidence wavered because I feared failure. Several attempts were complete failures, while others missed the mark but came close. I began to wonder if I would ever get back to normal. I had to dispel feelings of anger, discontent, and depression, and focus on the positive to be able to accomplish anything. I am very fortunate to have a loving patient wife who had helped me get through this. After about 7-8 months, I started having reasonably successful sex once a week, but I had love and intimacy every day. My wife and I enjoy a close relationship.

Something else happened. My dreams continued. I had recurrences of my ethereal out of body escape from the ICU, and my descent into the dark, sad void full of souls in a Purgatory-like state, where I escaped by following the light. I had new dreams where I found myself embracing a column of yellow flames that weren't hot, but instead felt like warm, intense peaceful light. Other people were behind me reaching toward it. I saw it a second time, and the column of light went up into the clouds where there were steps leading to an intense bright light radiating on a throne. I had a sense that a spiritual awakening was in process, and I felt peaceful about it.

In the months to follow, I continued writing the final chapters of this book and planned to do more art work. Another spring blossomed, and a blanket of pollen covered the entire city while I stayed inside and worked. Before long, the extremely hot summer surged into the calendar, while my recollections filled page after page. The book went forward, and so did my life.

CHAPTER EIGHT

THE MAGNITUDE OF SEPSIS

Knowledge is Power - Sir Francis Bacon, 1597

The seismic impact of sepsis shook me to the very core of my being. I was left trembling, hopeless, and nearly lifeless. My condition rapidly advanced to severe sepsis, becoming an internal earthquake of unexpected magnitude, overturning my life and challenging my will to live.

My near-death experience led me to further research about sepsis. I needed to know about the illness that became such an aggressive, destructive event in my life. This chapter is a brief look at the magnitude of sepsis, where I have tried to reduce an enormous amount of information into an overview that will hopefully ignite your curiosity, and spark your interest toward further reading and investigation about sepsis. Chances are that you know, or have heard about someone who has had sepsis or died from it, and statistics are a growing reminder that you probably will in the future. It is not a message of doom, but rather impending concern.

The worldwide rise of sepsis cases is grappling at the foundations of public health. Sepsis is shaking the medical world, creating a desperate need for ways to conquer this recalcitrant beast. The burden of sepsis is overwhelming, and reflected in high mortality rates, horrible suffering, great financial stress, and a debilitated quality of life for many of those who survive the ordeal. There are thousands of cases annually, and thousands of deaths, yet sepsis has not made its way into the American vocabulary.

Public Awareness

The majority of Americans are unfamiliar with sepsis, which causes one in four hospital deaths. This lack of awareness and understanding becomes a major challenge in healthcare. Lack of knowledge about the syndrome of sepsis may cause a patient to delay seeking medical care until late in the disease process. A survey done at the Feinstein Institute found that nearly 70 percent of adults 65 and older (who are particularly vulnerable) did not know what sepsis is, that the condition was least familiar to residents of Southern states, that more men than women were unfamiliar with sepsis (63 percent versus 55 percent), and that blacks were less familiar with the condition than whites and Hispanics. College graduates were found to have a greater understanding of sepsis than those who have no more than a high school education (50 percent versus 24 percent). The serious illness of sepsis remains something of an enigma to the general public (Feinstein Institute, 2010).

In an international survey of public awareness and perception of sepsis, 6021 interviewees, 5021 in Europe and 1000 in the United States were given structured telephone interviews. In Italy, Spain, the United Kingdom, France, and the United States a mean of 88% of interviewees had never heard of the term "sepsis". In Italy, Spain, the United Kingdom, France, and the United States, of people who recognized the term sepsis, 58% did not recognize that sepsis is a leading cause of death. These results show poor public awareness about the existence of a syndrome known as sepsis, and highlight the challenges of early management and treatment (Rubulotta, Ramsey, Parker, Dellinger, Levy, & Poeze, 2009). Since early detection and rapid accurate diagnosis and treatment are paramount in the management of sepsis, awareness of the signs and symptoms are of utmost importance in saving lives. *need a stroke-like campaign i.e. F-A-S-T*

Definitions and Symptoms

Sir William Osler, M.D. in "The Evolution of Modern Medicine" circa 1904 stated: "Except on few occasions, the patient appears to die from the body's response to infection rather than from it."(Opal, 2007).This is a key statement describing the syndrome of sepsis.

Sepsis is an enigmatic and complex syndrome with a broad range of clinical conditions caused by the body's response to an infection. It is an aggressive, multi-factorial, rapid killer. If it develops into severe sepsis, it can cause organ dysfunction or failure and death. The number of cases is increasing killing approximately 1,400 people worldwide every day (Society of Critical Care Medicine, 2002). While a definition and conceptual framework for sepsis is continuing to evolve, the process is widely thought of as a systemic inflammatory response syndrome (SIRS) triggered by an overwhelming infection. Severe sepsis occurs upon failure or dysfunction of at least one organ, and septic shock is defined by hypotension in the setting of severe sepsis, unresponsive to fluid resuscitation (Rello & Restreppo, 2008).

Sepsis is defined as a range of clinical conditions caused by the body's immune response to infection or trauma. This immune response is characterized by systemic (whole body) inflammation and disordered coagulation that can lead to organ failure or death. This syndrome can rapidly lead to loss of limbs, organ dysfunction, and ultimately death. The body's normal reaction to infection goes into overdrive, setting off a cascade of events that can lead to widespread inflammation and clotting.

As a medical term, sepsis refers to the evidence of an infection plus the presence of at least three of these criteria:

1. Heart rate greater than 90 beats/minute
2. Increased respiratory effort
3. High or low white blood cell count
4. Fever or low body temperature

Symptoms of sepsis may include reduced mental alertness, confusion, shaking, chills, fever, nausea, vomiting, and diarrhea in the presence of an infection (Eli Lilly and Company, 2010).

Sepsis results from the inability of the immune system to limit bacterial spread during an ongoing infection. Massive bacterial load overrides the inhibitory mechanisms controlling inflammation. While normally helping to eradicate pathogens from a local infection of peripheral tissues, inflammation during sepsis develops into a systemic syndrome, with multiple manifestations such as tissue injury, increased vascular permeability, and ultimately multi-organ failure and shock (Decker, 2004).

The systemic syndrome of sepsis was defined with the term systemic inflammatory response syndrome or SIRS by the American College of Chest Physicians and the Society of Critical Care Medicine at a conference in 1991. Sepsis was defined as the presence of infection plus SIRS.

The definition of SIRS was characterized by two or more of the following conditions:

1. Temperature higher than 38(degrees) C or lower than 36(degrees) C
2. Heart rate greater than 90 beats per minute
3. Respiratory rates greater than 20 breaths per minute
4. White blood cell count higher than 12,000 cells per micro liter or lower than 4,000 cells per micro liter

The goal of this consensus conference was to provide a conceptual and practical framework to define the systemic response to infection, and provide broad definitions that could improve the ability to make early bedside detection possible, thus allowing early therapeutic intervention. They offered detailed definitions for infection, bacteremia, septicemia, sepsis, severe sepsis, septic shock, hypotension, and multiple organ dysfunction. The systemic response to infection was termed sepsis; the systemic inflammatory response to a variety of insults was called SIRS, and severe sepsis would be associated with organ dysfunction, hypoperfusion, or hypotension (Bone, et al., 1992).

In 2001, an International Sepsis Definitions Conference was held to evaluate the strengths and weaknesses of the foundational definitions introduced in the 1991 consensus conference. Responding to medical research, they challenged the general definitions of sepsis and attempted to refine them, and offered a classification scheme and staging system for sepsis.

They concluded that current concepts of sepsis, severe sepsis, and septic shock were useful and remained unchanged, but the definitions did not allow precise characterization and staging of patients with these conditions. While SIRS remains a useful concept, diagnostic criteria published in 1992 was overly sensitive, nonspecific, and needed a more expanded list of signs and symptoms of sepsis to better reflect the clinical response to infection. The expanded diagnostic criteria included the following parameters: general, inflammatory, hemodynamic, organ dysfunction, and tissue perfusion.

They developed a classification scheme for sepsis called PIRO, that stratifies patients on the basis of their Predisposing conditions, Insult (in the case of sepsis, infection), the nature and magnitude of the host Response, and the degree of concomitant Organ dysfunction. This staging system became the ground work for more extensive testing and further refinement (Levy, et al., 2003). Both of these seminal conferences and reports helped pave the way for the development and implementation of working definitions for sepsis and SIRS which have been globally adopted by clinicians and investigators, as well as generating models for future research.

Sepsis can generate a wide variety of symptoms. Some of the most prominent are: decreased urine output, fast heart rate (tachycardia), fever (high body temperature), hypothermia (very low body temperature), shaking, chills, warm skin or a skin rash, confusion or delirium, and hyperventilation (rapid breathing). Common sites of infection that can lead to sepsis include the abdomen, the lungs, the skin, the central nervous system, and the urinary tract (Cleveland Clinic, 2010).

Sepsis is extremely dangerous, and can originate anywhere in the body. It can be subtle, rapid, and often deadly, progressing from an initial inflammation from a variety of causes such as trauma, burns, surgical sites, intravenous lines, recent or long term illness, or myocardial infarction to a systemic inflammatory response syndrome (SIRS). As certain criteria are met, such as a temperature higher than 38 degrees C (100.4 F), or lower than 36 degrees C (96.8 F), and heart rate greater than 90 beats per minute, the sepsis progression escalates toward severe sepsis with signs and symptoms of organ failure that can be cardiovascular, neurologic, pulmonary, and renal. At this point, aggressive treatment is required in a critical care area to prevent septic shock and death (Nelson, LeMaster, Plost,& Zahner,2009).

Sepsis is an enigmatic, insidious, under-recognized condition which is the leading cause of death in non-cardiac ICUs (intensive care units). Symptoms can be subtle and progress over time without obvious indicators. It can develop in lethal obscurity, and without vigilant attention may be recognized too late, limiting effectiveness of available treatments (Ahrens, 2007).

The sepsis syndrome is unpredictable, and diagnosing sepsis can be complicated. Symptoms such as fever, rapid pulse, and respiratory difficulty are very general and mimic many other disorders. A patient may quickly deteriorate into septic shock or suffer from organ dysfunction, and in up to 30 percent of cases a definite source of infection cannot be identified (Eli Lilly and Company, 2010).

In my own case, sepsis was a barely noticed subtle progression, and I did not go to the doctor right away. I thought I had a sinus infection with a mild fever and self-treated at home, but the bomb was about to explode, and I didn't know it. I also did not really know what sepsis was, or the signs and symptoms. I can assure you that I do now. I repeatedly asked the doctors about the source of my infection, and they could not identify it. The lab work was inconclusive, and the mystery remains.

With sepsis, a patient's overwhelming response to infection or invading microorganisms becomes his own worst enemy that triggers a dangerous cascade of events that become an unregulated and uncontrolled auto-destructive process. The bacterial infection over-stimulates the body's immune system, setting off a cascade of inflammatory and abnormal clotting responses that can lead to organ failure and death. The pathophysiology of sepsis can be the result of infection at any body site, and can be initiated by gram-positive or gram-negative organisms as well as fungal, viral, and parasitic invading organisms.

Severe sepsis is associated with three integrated responses: activation of inflammation, activation of coagulation, and impaired fibrinolysis. These three responses become responsible for and contribute to impaired tissue function and organ damage. This imbalance between inflammation, coagulation, and fibrinolysis (breakdown of clots) that occurs in severe sepsis results in systemic inflammation, widespread coagulopathy (abnormal clotting), and macrovascular thrombosis, conditions which can lead to multiple organ dysfunction and death. Severe sepsis is associated with an unacceptable mortality rate of 28% to 50% (Kleinpell, 2003).

Under normal circumstances, the body's defense system releases immune modulators to help fight infection and heal itself. But in severe sepsis, the process breaks down, and immune modulators go into overdrive. This sets off a cascade of events that can lead to widespread inflammation and blood clotting in tiny vessels throughout the body. The clots can form in vital organs, arms, legs, and digits, limiting blood flow and causing tissue damage, which can lead to organ failure, loss of limbs, and death (Hopper, 2009).

The complex interplay between activation of excessive inflammation and coagulation with impaired fibrinolysis in sepsis continues to be a challenge for research and development. The Eli Lilly and Company product called Xygris (drotrecogin alfa (activated) or recombinant human activated Protein C has emerged after years of research as the only drug with proven efficacy in treating life-threatening severe sepsis, with a 29% relative risk reduction in patients at a higher risk of death. This activated Protein C is an important mechanism for regulating inflammation, coagulation and fibrinolysis (Eli Lilly and Company, 2010).

It is hard to imagine having an infection that quickly unfolds into a lethal and insidious inflammatory response syndrome, where your own immune system turns against you killing cells and shutting down organs. You can die from your own body's response to infection, rather from the infection itself.

Studies, Incidence, and Outcome

Epidemiology is the study of incidence, distribution, and control of disease in a population (Novartis Diagnostics Global, 2010). Data is collected from samples that are representative of a population about sepsis related illness and deaths to build a body of knowledge that serves as a foundation and logic of interventions made in the interest of public health and preventative medicine (Wikipedia Encyclopedia, 2010). These samples vary in size and are researched with major characteristic variables in person, time, and place, such as geographic location, race and ethnic breakdown, short and long term studies, and trends (Videojug Corporation, 2010). This data can include population-based health registries, medical records, national health surveys, and other public health systems which help to study the course or history of disease, determine the frequency of disease in populations, identify the patterns of disease occurrence, identify risk factors for and potential causes of disease, and evaluate the effectiveness of preventative and treatment measures. Findings have the potential to influence governments, public health agencies, and medical organizations policies and practices, and also create and stimulate public awareness (Autism Speaks, 2010).

Studies vary on incidence and outcome concerning sepsis, and there are disparities (such as comorbidities) that can change the percentages, but most important is the fact that sepsis is a growing worldwide problem. I am now a statistic in the ever-mounting list of severe sepsis cases, but fortunately not in the mortality rates.

The studies I have included show the burden of sepsis, and have helped to set off the alarm in the United States and other countries around the world. These are just a few examples, and are much more detailed and elaborate than this chapter can contain.

In a significant epidemiology to determine the incidence, cost, and outcome of severe sepsis in the United States, Dr. Derek C. Angus and colleagues (2001) linked all 1995 state hospital discharge records in seven states forming an enormous patient database which was supplemented with hospital and population data from the U.S. Census Bureau, the Centers for Disease Control, the Health Care Financing Administration, and the American Hospital Association. Severe sepsis was defined as documented infection and acute organ dysfunction. They identified 192,980 patients with severe sepsis. After adjustment for age and gender, statistical analysis produced a national incidence estimate of 3.0 cases per 1,000 population, or 751,000 cases annually. The overall hospital mortality rate was 28.6% or 215,000 deaths annually nationwide, with mortality increasing with age. They concluded that severe sepsis is a common, expensive, and frequently fatal condition, with as many deaths annually as those from acute myocardial infarction, and that it is especially common in the elderly and is likely to increase as the population ages. Total costs for severe sepsis were estimated to be $16.7 billion, at an average cost per case of $22,100 (Angus, et al., 2001). Dr. Angus and his colleagues project that the incidence of sepsis will increase by 1.5% per year, mostly attributed to the high incidence of sepsis in the elderly, and the overall aging of the population. They estimate that there will be 934,000 cases in the United States in the year 2010 and 1,110,000 cases in 2020 (Pulmonary Reviews, 2001).

Another important long –term study done by Dr. Greg S. Martin and colleagues (2003), investigated the epidemiology of sepsis in the United States from 1979 through 2000 examining race and sex, causative organisms, the disposition of patients, and the incidence and outcome. They reviewed discharge data on approximately 750 million hospitalizations over the 22-year period and identified 10,319,418 cases of sepsis. The average age of patients with sepsis increased consistently over time, from 57.4 years in the first sub-period to 60.8 years in the last sub-period. The four sub-periods were: 1979 through 1984, 1985 through 1989, 1990 through 1994, and 1995 through 2000. Sepsis developed later in life in female patients than in male patients. The mean age among women was 62.1 years as compared with 56.9 years among men.

Between 1979 and 2000 there was an annualized increase in the incidence of sepsis of 8.7 percent, from about 164,000 cases to nearly 660,000 cases. The rate of sepsis due to fungal organisms increased 207 percent, with gram-positive bacteria becoming the predominant pathogens after 1987. Sepsis was more common among men than women and among non-white persons than among white persons. Black men had the highest rate of sepsis, the youngest age at onset (mean age 47.4 years), and the highest mortality (23.3 percent

cent). In-hospital mortality rates declined over the 22-year period from 27.8 percent to 17.9 percent, but despite the improved survival rates, the incidence of sepsis and the number of sepsis-related deaths increased to nearly a tripling the number of in-hospital deaths related to sepsis from 43,579 deaths in 1979 to 120,491 deaths in 2000.

They indicated that care of patients with sepsis costs as much as $50,000 per patient with an economic burden of $17 billion annually in the United States. Possible reasons for the increased incidence of sepsis were: the increased use of invasive procedures and immunosuppressive drugs, chemo-therapy, and transplantation; the emergence of the epidemic of the human immune deficiency virus (HIV) infection, and increasing microbial resistance. The substantial increase in the incidence of sepsis during the past 22 years has placed sepsis among the 10 leading causes of death in the United States (Martin, Mannino, Eaton & Moss, 2003).

Dombrovsky and colleagues (2007) used discharge data from the Nationwide Inpatients Sample that is a 20% stratified sample of all U.S. community hospitals to conduct a trend analysis study in rates of hospitalization, mortality and hospital case fatality for severe sepsis in the United States for the period from 1993 to 2003. Using subjects of any age with sepsis including severe sepsis who were hospitalized in the United States during the study period they identified 8,403,766 patients with sepsis, including 2,857,476 patients with severe sepsis. The percentage of severe sepsis cases increased continuously from 25.6% in 1993 to 43.8% in 2003. During each year of the study the rates of hospitaliza-tion, mortality, and case fatality increased with age. They stated that the rate of severe sepsis almost doubled during the 11-year period studied, and was much greater than previous predictions. Mortality from severe sepsis increased significantly while case fatality rates decreased by 1.4%. Hospitalization and mortality rates in males exceeded those in females, but case fatality rate was greater in females (Dombrovsky, Martin, Sunderram & Paz, 2007).

Melamed and Sorvillo (2009) analyzed multiple-cause-of-death data from the National Center for Health Statistics from 1999 to 2005 to investigate trends, assess disparities, and provide population-based estimates of sepsis-associated mortality in the United States. They analyzed age, sex, race, ethnicity, year of death, place-of-death, and any other medical conditions mentioned on the death certificate. They found that 6% of all deaths in the United States from 1995 to 2005 were sepsis related, and that only 22.7% of sepsis-associated deaths would be attributed to sepsis using the underlying-cause-of-death classification. This classification may contribute to significantly underestimating the true burden of sepsis-associated mortality, because in patients who had underlying pathologies or comorbidities, sepsis may not be listed as the underlying cause of death. For example, in cases where sepsis resulted from a nosocomial (hospital acquired) infection, the original reason for the hospitalization, rather than the sepsis is often listed as the underlying cause of death. They found significant racial disparities in sepsis-associated mortality. After controlling for age, Asians were less likely to experience sepsis-related death, while Blacks, American Indians/Alaska Natives and Hispanics were more likely to experience sepsis-related death. Young children and the elderly experienced the greatest burden of sepsis-related

Allison's post-abdominal Sx sepsis @ age 12!

death. The researchers concluded that the rapid rise in sepsis mortality seen in previous decades has slowed, but population aging continues to drive growth in the burden of sepsis-associated mortality. Sepsis continues to be a major contributor to mortality in the United States, and is a 10th leading cause of death (Melamed & Sorvillo, 2009).

The results of a literature review of the epidemiology of sepsis in Latin America suggest that the clinical and epidemiological approaches to the problem of sepsis have sometimes been inappropriate in research design, study population, and clinical outcome. Some data suggested that in terms of both frequency and mortality the situation with sepsis and severe systemic infections may be worse in Latin America than it is in developed countries. Higher mortality rates indicate a growing problem and require increased public and professional awareness of high frequency and mortality associated with sepsis, and early and accurate diagnosis of sepsis by developing a clear and clinically relevant definition of sepsis (Jaimes, 2005).

Other countries are contributing to the magnitude of sepsis, making it a world-wide problem. Shen, Lu, and Yang (2010) analyzed the hospital claims data of a nationally representative sample of 200,000 people, which is approximately 1 percent of the population enrolled in their Taiwan National Health Insurance Program. Their study examined the epidemiologic trend of severe sepsis in Taiwan from 1997 through 2006. They identified first and subsequent episodes in 5,258 patients having 7,531 hospitalizations for severe sepsis during a 10-year period and concluded that the incidence and severity of severe sepsis in Taiwan are increasing. The proportion of patients with multi-organ dysfunctions increased from 11.7% to 27.6%. The hospital mortality rate changed little, averaging 30.8%, and among survivors, 34.4% developed at least one more subsequent severe sepsis episode (Shen & Lu, 2010).

In a study involving ninety-one general intensive care units in England, Wales, and Northern Ireland between 1995 and 2000, researchers found that 27.1% of adult intensive care unit admissions met severe sepsis criteria in the first 24 hours in the intensive care unit. Of the intensive care admissions that met the severe sepsis criteria in the first 24 hours, 35% died before intensive care unit discharge, and 47% died during their hospital stay (Padkin, et al., 2003).

A study by the Episepsis group surveyed patients with severe sepsis in 206 French ICUs over two consecutive weeks in 2001. The mean age of the patients was 65 years, and 54.1% had at least one chronic organ system dysfunction (comorbid condition). Mortality was 35% at 30 days; at 2 months the mortality rate was 41.9%, and 11.4% of patients remained hospitalized. Ten years ago 8.4% of patients in French intensive care units were found to have severe sepsis or shock with a 56% mortality rate in the hospital. In this study 14.6% of patients experienced severe sepsis or shock with a lower overall mortality rate. The incidence of severe sepsis appears to have increased but associated mortality has decreased, possibly due to implementation of newer therapies or effective management strategies (Brun-Buisson, Meshaka, Pinton & Vallet, 2004).

A severe sepsis study was conducted in 12 intensive therapy units (ITUs) in India from June 2006 to November 2006 to determine the incidence and outcome of severe sepsis among adult patients. A total of 1,344 ITU admissions were studied. The mean age of the population was 54.9 years, of which 67% were male, and the incidence of severe sepsis was 13.1% of all admissions. ITU mortality of all admissions was 13.9%, and that of severe sepsis was 54.1%. Hospital mortality and 28-day mortality of severe sepsis were 59.3% and 57.6% (Todi, Chatterjee & Bhattacharyya, 2007).

Another study conducted in four intensive therapy units (ITUs) in India from June 2006 to June 2009. A total of 5,478 ITU admissions were studied. The mean age of the population was 58.17 years, of which 57.71% were male, and the incidence of severe sepsis was 16.45% of all admissions. All patients were screened daily for SIRS, organ dysfunction and severe sepsis. The ITU mortality of all admissions was 12.08% and that of severe sepsis was 59.26%. Hospital mortality and 28-day mortality of severe sepsis were 65.2% and 64.6%. Gram-negative organisms were responsible for 72.45% of cases and gram-positive for 13.3%. The rest were parasitic, viral, and fungal infections (Todi, Chatterjee, Shu & Bhattacharyya, 2010).

Severe sepsis was common in Indian ITUs with a high mortality rate, and gram-negative organisms were predominant. Todi points out that awareness of sepsis as a disease entity is poor among the general population and the physician community. With hardly any public demand for research in this field, the progress of science has been limited. There is a critical need to disseminate awareness to expand the horizons of sepsis (Todi, 2010).

An epidemiology of sepsis was completed in Victoria, Australia utilizing hospital discharge data of 3,122,515 overnight hospitalizations over a 4-year period from July 1, 1999 to June 30, 2003. The main results indicated that the overall hospital incidence of sepsis was 1.1%, with a mortality of 18.4%. Of septic patients, 23.8% received care in an ICU. These patients had a hospital mortality of 28.9% Severe sepsis, which was defined by sepsis and at least one organ dysfunction, occurred in 39% of sepsis patients, with a hospital mortality of 31.3%. Incidence and outcome were similar to reports from comparable populations in North America and Europe (Sundararajan, Macisaac, Presneill, Cade & Visvanathan, 2005).

In 2009, the Canadian Institute for Health Information released a report focused upon a national picture of sepsis hospitalizations and mortality. In 2008-2009, 30,587 sepsis hospitalizations were observed in Canada (outside Quebec) and 9,320 sepsis patients died. The crude mortality rate for all sepsis patients was high at 30.5%, 45.2% for severe sepsis, and 20.9% for patients whose sepsis did not progress to severe. Older adults and young children accounted for the majority of sepsis case with patients 60 and older comprising 60.6% of all hospitalizations in 2008-2009. Among these patients, 54.6% were men, while 44.5% were women. Sepsis patients tended to have more pre-existing comorbidities, with 44.5% having at least one comorbidity. Factors contributing to a higher chance of dying were being older, being female (8% higher odds), having pre-admission comorbidities, having sepsis occurring after admission to the hospital, and having severe sepsis. Severe sepsis patients had about three times higher odds of dying than patients whose sepsis was not severe. Overall, 5,447, or 58.4% of sepsis patients who died had severe sepsis. The burden of sepsis has continued to grow. Canadian hospitals continue their efforts to refine early identification and treatment, and heighten the general awareness and understanding of sepsis as a step toward reducing mortality rates (Canadian Institute for Health Information, 2009).

Quality of Life

What happens to sepsis survivors? Are they able to resume a normal life? What are the far-reaching effects that extend beyond hospitalization? Some survivors live normal lives again, others recover but with limitations and challenges, and some are devastated in the aftermath.

Quartin and his colleagues were the first to show that sepsis has long-lasting effects and increases the risk of death up to 5 years after hospitalization for the septic episode. Within one year of surviving sepsis, there is a 26% predicted mortality rate. The risk of death during the first year is associated with the severity of the septic episode (Quartin, Schein, Kett & Peduzzi, 1997).

Although sepsis is a deadly, acute disease, survivors also suffer long-term consequences. The septic population is at significant risk of dying of non-septic causes for up to 8 years after the initial hospitalization. The initial severe response sets in motion a dysregulated immune/inflammatory response which has long-lasting implications regarding how someone responds to and deals with other challenges. Alterations on a cellular level from the acute disease of sepsis can result in immunosuppression, which can lead to secondary infection, and increase the risk of death. The chronic consequences of severe sepsis can produce an impaired quality of life after surviving the initial challenge (Benjamin, Hogaboam, & Kunkel, 2004).

Long-term mortality following sepsis is high, and fewer than half of patients who experience severe sepsis are alive at 1 year. Studies suggest that abnormalities of the innate immune system may contribute to increased long-term mortality. Mechanisms underlying increased long-term mortality remain poorly understood (Yende & Angus, 2007).

Prolonged recovery after severe sepsis can lead to a core of physical and psychological problems that need interventions through rehabilitation. Physical problems can include severe muscle wasting, weight loss, and degeneration of motor nerves, which can lead to poor muscle strength, fatigue causing difficulties that require help with feeding, walking or climbing stairs. Psychological issues can include anxiety, depression, post-traumatic stress disorder, agoraphobia, and panic attacks. Stress disorders may be precipitated from delusional memories of hallucinations, nightmares, or paranoid delusions recalled from time in the ICU. An idea originated in Sweden makes use of ICU diaries as therapy to reduce impact of delusional memories and establish rebuilding memories of events in the ICU. Significant cognitive deficits may have an impact on the ability of patients to achieve care for themselves (Jones & Griffiths, 2006).

In my own case, I was very fortunate to having a loving, caring family that helped me "reconnect" with reality on a daily basis. They re-explained procedures that were done in the ICU when I was confused or delirious. They spoke softly

what's the impact of or no visitors on these pts?

115

and kindly to me, and prayed for me. After every visit they wrote "we were here" on the chalkboard in my room, with a list of everyone that visited that day. Love lifted me.

A long-term follow up study of the impact of severe sepsis on health-related quality of life showed that patients surviving sepsis can have an impaired quality of life. After sharp declines during their ICU stay, gradual improvement occurred during the following six months, but despite survival, recovery was incomplete in physical functioning, role-physical, and general health dimensions compared with the situation before the ICU stay. Sepsis had a significant impact on long-term outcomes (Hofhuis, et al., 2008).

A long-term study was done in Finland in 24 ICUs of adult patients with severe sepsis. They concluded that the two-year mortality after severe sepsis was high at 44.9%. and that the quality of life was lower after severe sepsis than before critical illness (Karlsson, Ruokonen, Varpula, Ala-Kokko & Pettila, 2009).

A systematic review of studies reporting long-term mortality and quality of life data in patients with sepsis, severe sepsis, and septic shock showed that sepsis survivors consistently demonstrated impaired quality of life. Results were consistent across varying severity of illness and different patient populations in different countries, including large and small studies (Winters, et al., 2020).

Besides the high mortality rate associated with sepsis, studies have shown that ICU survivors present long-term cognitive impairment, including alterations in memory, attention, concentration, and/or global loss of cognitive function. The pathogenesis of septic encephalopathy and cognitive impairment is still poorly known, and further knowledge of these processes is necessary for the development of effective preventive and therapeutic treatment (Comim, et al., 2009).

In a survey of survivors of septic illness and acute myocardial infarction(control group), individuals in the sepsis group reported more symptoms on the sensory, physical, and behavior sections of the questionnaire form. They had greater difficulty with sleep and rest, emotional behavior, body care and movement, and physical and psychosocial functioning. Other symptoms included problem solving, concentration, memory, and sensory and physical ability. These problems become most apparent when involved in challenging activities, such as working (Lazosky, Young, Zirul & Phillips, 2009).

Cognitive impairment and functional disability are substantial and persistent among survivors of severe sepsis. All is not normal once the infection is better. Many elderly survivors of severe sepsis return home after hospital discharge with major new deficits in their ability to live independently. In a study examining disability and cognitive outcomes among 516 survivors of severe sepsis with an average age of 77 years, they averaged 1.5 new functional limitations compared to their pre-sepsis baseline. These limitations have a profound effect on the ability to live independently. Problems included requiring help of a care giver to manage finances, take medicine, bathe, or get dressed (Iwashyna, Ely, Smith & Langa, 2010). The post-discharge care for elders is a growing concern as it becomes a potential geriatric nightmare. *everything is a geriatric nightmare !!*

117

Other studies have recommended that future studies in patients with severe sepsis should include long-term follow up throughout hospitalization and after hospital discharge. Long-term focus on quality of life (QoL) should be concerned with physical, psychological, and social functioning, and should include objective assessments and the patient's subjective experiences to determine therapeutic needs relevant to restoring the ability to function on a daily basis (Rublee, Opal, Schramm, Keinecke & Knaub, 2002).

The Ohio State University Sepsis Registry is an ongoing observational study designed to collect follow-up information about patients with sepsis in the Ohio State University Medical Center (OSUMC) MICU who survive to hospital discharge. The study started in December, 2006, and has an estimated completion date of February, 2012. Specific aims are to collect follow-up information about sepsis patients, collect a registry of patients who would be interested in hearing more information about future prospective studies for survivors of sepsis, and to collect a blood sample from admitted patients for future retrospective IRB-approved studies. These goals will provide information for future studies, and by following survivors of sepsis for a prolonged period, they will better understand the disease process and the duration of recovery (Ohio State University Sepsis Registry, 2009).

The purpose of a recent study, the international PROGRESS (Promoting Global Research Excellence in Severe Sepsis) registry of patients with severe sepsis was to compare baseline characteristics and clinical outcomes of patients treated or not treated with drotrecogin alfa activated (DrotAA;

recombinant human protein C). This global study, involving 37 countries and 12,492 patients, is one of the largest severe sepsis registries to date. It was developed and designed with the intervention of documentary profiles of disease diagnosis (epidemiologic, etiologic, and baseline severity data), patient management, and outcomes in real-life clinical settings across several regions of the world (Martin, et al., 2009).

There is an entire curriculum that needs to be developed for sepsis survivors after discharge from the hospital. It would go beyond the basics, with a design to achieve a return to normal in every aspect of impairment that sepsis patients endure. Goals and objectives need to be developed to meet this growing need, and must be coordinated with the most recent research. Successful implementation would require patient needs assessments, specialized post-discharge rehab programs, and guidelines that go beyond the basics of self-care. As sepsis is studied further, rehab interventions can be refined to meet the needs of those patients who survive sepsis, and produce a better quality of life.

Fourteen months after returning home from the hospital, I still tire easily after doing everyday tasks, and I really fade after doing harder tasks like waxing a car or sanding a table to refinish it. Some muscles are still a little weaker than they used to be, and my stamina is slightly reduced. It can take up to two days to feel back to normal. I am more emotional at times when reacting to conflicts, tragedy, or stressful situations. I cry more often, and I don't always know why. Sometimes, I have flashbacks to the ICU when I was nearing death, or to the black Purgatory-like room of anguish. I have greater skin sensitivity since my body was so stretched and swollen back in the ICU. A flare-up of the scabies on my fingers led to a swollen hand and wrist, and I had to get a cortisone shot and Prednisone tablets to recover from it. This may be evidence that severe sepsis affected my immune system and has made me more vulnerable. I also heal much slower from insect bites, cuts, rashes, and abrasions than I did prior to having sepsis. I have gotten over most of my anxiety and depression, although I do wonder at times just how much longer I have to live. Overall, I feel reasonably normal with a renewed spirit writing this book and doing art work that has become part of my rehabilitation and sense of purpose.

Sepsis Losses

Many brave and courageous individuals have overcome a myriad of difficult challenges in their post-sepsis aftermath, and give others hope and inspiration. There are also many stories about loss. These are just a few that have fallen victim to sepsis and died.

Christopher Reeve, actor, film director, screenwriter, and author died of sepsis in 2004 at age 52. He became a quadriplegic after being thrown from a horse in 1995, and lived in a wheel chair with a breathing apparatus for the rest of his life. He was well known as the star of the motion picture Superman. He died of sepsis from a bed sore that became infected and spread into his bloodstream, becoming a systemic infection, which he had experienced many times before. He went into cardiac arrest after receiving an antibiotic for the infection and fell into a coma, dying soon afterward (Bookofjoe, 2004).

Jim Henson, famous puppeteer and creator of The Muppets, died of septic shock and organ failure at age 53. On May 4th, 1990 he had flu-like symptoms. Later on May 12th he felt tired and sick with no evidence of pneumonia after a doctor's exam. By May 15th he had trouble breathing and went to the hospital and died the next day May 16th, 1990 from organ failure (Wikipedia Encyclopedia, 2010).

Mariana Bridi da Costa, Brazilian model, died on January 24th, 2009, at 20 years old. She was first diagnosed as suffering from a urinary infection, but by the time it was detected it had developed into septicemia. The sepsis caused insufficient blood flow, and she developed necrosis, septic shock, and organ failure. Her body was ravaged by the disease and doctors performed amputations of her hands and feet, and extracted part of her stomach and both kidneys in a desperate attempt to save her. The sepsis cascade exploded rapidly and killed her at age 20. Prior to her hospitalization, and unfortunate and sad death, she was a vibrant young woman, well on her way to achieving her dreams as a world-class model (Whiteman & deMoura, 2009).

In 2002, 23 year-old Erin Flatley of Dunedin, Florida went into the hospital for a minor hemorrhoid procedure, and less than a week later died a horrible death from sepsis. Soon after she returned home, from minor surgery, she was in serious pain. Two days after surgery she was taken to the emergency room where they noticed an elevated white blood cell count, but hesitated to start her on antibiotics, and sent her home with a topical cream. Her pain was excruciating and she had trouble urinating and was taken back to the hospital and eventually prescribed antibiotics which were delayed in being administered. She was shaking and thrashing in her bed with a high heart rate and low blood pressure. The cascade of sepsis brought her into septic shock, and she died the next morning just six days after surgery (Thompson, 2005). Erin's father, Dr. Carl Flatley has a made difference out of her memory by founding the Sepsis Alliance, which is a public charity dedicated to the early detection, effective management, and cure of sepsis worldwide (Flatley, 2002).

The word sepsis is derived from the Greek word sepein, meaning "to rot". The mention of it appeared in the poems of Homer, the Greek epic poet more than 2700 years ago (Chang, Lynm & Glass, 2010). Sepsis has been weaving its way throughout history ever since.

A quick glance at the Civil War in the United States back in the 1860's indicates the presence of sepsis during an era before antiseptic surgery, where sterility was not considered necessary and this caused more infections and mortality. Battlefield wounds often became infected which led to sepsis, a systemic with a mortality rate of more than 90%. Many amputations were performed to prevent sepsis and reduce mortality rates to 20-25 percent. Sepsis played a tragic part of the Civil War (Wheat, 2010).

Years later in 1881, James A. Garfield, 20th President of the United States was shot in the back by an assassin and suffered for 80 days until he died. Although he officially died from his wound, which was considered a non-lethal injury, many believe that his surgeons killed him by probing the wound with unwashed hands and unwashed silver probes trying to locate and extract the bullet. Garfield's doctors introduced terrible infections through this repeated probing, spreading bacteria causing him to suffer from fever spikes and rigors. His autopsy revealed multiple pus cavities, and it was determined that he died of sepsis and starvation (Herr, 2007).

Sepsis Organizations

Various forums, groups, symposiums, and alliances are addressing the need for greater understanding and management of sepsis. Doctors and researchers are very aware of the increasing incidence of sepsis cases and associated high mortality rates throughout the world. They have combined their efforts to improve the treatment of sepsis and reduce the high mortality rates. The following are a few examples that represent the dedicated efforts against the growing epidemic of sepsis.

The Surviving Sepsis Campaign is a global initiative to bring together professional organizations in reducing mortality from sepsis. This international collaborative effort was developed by the European Society of Critical Care Medicine, the International Sepsis Forum, and the Society of Critical Care Medicine, to help meet the challenges of sepsis and improve its management, diagnosis, and treatment. The overall goal of the campaign is to increase clinician and public awareness of the incidence of sepsis, severe sepsis, and septic shock, to develop guidelines for the management of severe sepsis, and to foster a change in the standard of care in sepsis management.

The campaign was initiated in 2002 and implemented in three phases. The first phase introduced the campaign in Barcelona, Spain where they announced a target of 25 percent reduction in mortality from severe sepsis over the next five years. The second phase aimed at producing guidelines for the management of sepsis with a conference held in Windsor, UK where they conducted a thorough evidence-based review of the literature in both diagnosis and manage-ment of infection, and the management of sepsis. The confe-rence resulted in the establishment of a series of guidelines for the management of sepsis. Phase three, in 2008, aimed to operationalize the guidelines and transform them into user-friendly tools to implement into bedside care. These were landmark publications that began a global standard of care for sepsis management (Society of Critical Care Medicine, 2002). Guidelines were made into operational "bundles" to implement resuscitation and management for the first 6 hours after recognition as well as a 24 hour bundle to follow, which establishes an evidence-based standard of care and facilitates knowledge transfer to the bedside of critically ill septic patients (Parker, 2010).

The Surviving Sepsis Campaign has saved lives, facilitated knowledge, and established an improved standard of care for septic patients around the world. As an example, through implementation of the Surviving Sepsis Campaign guidelines at three medical-surgical intensive care units of an academic tertiary care center, a significant decrease in mortality was accomplished. In-hospital mortality was reduced from 57.3% to 37.5% (Castellanos-Ortega, 2010).

The International Sepsis Forum (ISF) is a collaborative effort between industry and academia, and is the first initiative to focus solely on management of patients with severe sepsis. It was launched in 1997, and is now a multi-sponsored group supported by unrestricted education grants from pharmaceutical and diagnostic companies, along with donations from the general public. Their Guidelines for the Management of Severe Sepsis and Septic Shock were published in 2001 and used as a starting point for guidelines developed by the Surviving Sepsis Campaign. Their vision is to reduce global morbidity and mortality from sepsis. Their mission is to improve the care of critical care patients with sepsis by promoting an improved understanding of the basic biology and pathology of sepsis, to enhance understanding of the epidemiology of sepsis, to improve design and conduct of clinical research, to educate health professionals in optimal management, and to raise the profile of sepsis as a global health challenge with the public, healthcare practitioners, industry, and global health agencies.

In 2010, they held an International Symposium at the Institut Pasteur, Paris, France where they addressed topics like the Global Burden of Sepsis, refining the Treatment of Sepsis, trials and research, as well as the pathogenesis of sepsis. Delegates left the symposium with greater understanding of sepsis from molecular, biochemistry, and physiology perspectives through to clinical management of the septic patient. The next Symposium will be held in October, 2011 at the China National Convention Center, Beijing, China (International Sepsis Forum, 2010).

Other organizations include the German Sepsis Society (GSS), the Global Sepsis Alliance, and the Sepsis Alliance. There are several other groups, but there isn't room in this chapter to include them all.

The German Sepsis Society's mission is to educate and increase public and professional awareness about sepsis. They have developed guidelines for prevention, diagnosis, therapy and follow-up care of sepsis. This medical society organizes public activities and medical training, and has established a research platform that will help to improve diagnosis of sepsis and identification of patients at risk, advance the understanding of the pathophysiology of sepsis, evaluate novel therapeutic approaches of sepsis, improve treatment, and investigate epidemiology and conduct health economic assessments of sepsis. They also support lobbying for sepsis by targeting funding agencies and health policy makers (German Sepsis Society, 2010).

The Global Sepsis Alliance (GSA) is a new collaboration of the World Federation of Societies of Intensive and Critical Care Medicine, the World Federation of Pediatric Intensive and Critical Care Societies, the International Sepsis Forum, and the Sepsis Alliance. The objective of the Global Sepsis Alliance is to rally the global sepsis community in an effort to elevate public, philanthropic, and government awareness, understanding and support of sepsis, and to accelerate collaboration among researchers, clinicians, and associated working groups and those dedicated to supporting them. The GSA is urging healthcare providers, patients, and policy makers worldwide to treat sepsis as a medical emergency. Sepsis is an enormous public health problem reaching epidemic proportions, and a global initiative is needed to reduce the mortality rate through consensus of definition, awareness, and application of diagnostic and treatment protocols for sepsis (Global Sepsis Alliance, 2010).

A recent international call to action was the Merinoff Symposium, September 29-October 1, 2010 in Manhasset, New York, hosted by the Feinstein Institute for medical research (Global Sepsis Alliance, 2010). This was a historic event in the field of sepsis, with goals to produce a current molecular definition of sepsis, a public definition of sepsis, and to issue a call-to-action to recognize sepsis as the leading cause of death worldwide (Merinoff Symposia, 2010).

The Sepsis Alliance was founded by Dr. Carl J. Flatley. His daughter Erin was a victim of sepsis. Her horrible and tragic death became the driving force that initiated the formation of the Sepsis Alliance. Dr. Flatley has made sepsis awareness, early detection, and effective management his personal mission and professional pursuit. The Sepsis Alliance is a charitable organization run by a team of dedicated lay people and professionals who share a strong commitment to battling sepsis. They are dedicated to the deployment of a global system supporting education, early recognition, and effective treatment, with a core mission to connect patients, families, and medical professionals with the tools to successfully combat sepsis (Sepsis Alliance, 2002).

All of these organizations are waging a battle against sepsis, which is under-recognized and poorly understood. It is an arduous task that requires massive medical synergy to become effective.

Sepsis Research

Yet, the sepsis monster continues to terrify and devour its victims at an alarming rate. No panacea exists for sepsis, but research continues to address early detection and diagnosis, and accurate, timely treatment, and management. Here are a few significant and interesting developments and advances in sepsis research.

The biotech firm MedaSorb is testing its medical device Cytosorb which is patented for its usage as a blood purificator. It removes toxins from the blood, allowing recirculation of clean blood back into the body. The device filters the blood for so called cytokines which are over-produced by the immune system and cause a toxic state in the body causing damage to cells, tissues, and organs. Trial phases have begun with hope to gain approval soon for launching it commercially. This may be a significant product in the fight against sepsis (Carsten, 2010).

In the UK, a research team in the school of Pharmacy and Biomolecular Sciences is working with the company Mast Carbon, two other universities, and a hospital, creating, testing, and producing a carbon filter with very small pores that traps specific biomolecules. The patient's blood can be pumped through a machine containing the filter and back into the body. The filter can also remove endotoxins which are damaging fragments left behind when bacteria that caused the original infection were attacked by the patient's immune system. Through efficient removal of cytokines and endotoxins, sepsis may be successfully treated (University of Brighton, 2010).

Scientists at Children's Hospital Boston are developing a miniature filtration device that can rapidly pump blood out of the body, clearing it of infectious agents before delivering the blood back to the body. It can be used in combination with antibiotics as a first line of defense treating sepsis before the antibiotics take effect. The prototype is designed in theory after the spleen. This blood filter, for microfiltering sepsis, uses a small magnetic field with specific molecules coated with tiny magnetic beads in solution that draw pathogens out of the blood. It is still in the development stage, with goals of incorporating the microfluidic device into a cartridge form, which can be snapped into any conventional hemofiltration or dialysis system (Chu, 2008).

Ming-Yie Lu and Dur-Zong Hsu at the Department of Environmental and Occupational Health, National Cheng Kung University in Taiwan found that one single dose of sesame oil had significant protection against sepsis. The main antioxidative component obtained from the sesame oil is called sesamol, which has delayed mortality and attenuated hepatic injury in rats which were induced with sepsis by cecal legation and puncture. Sesamol has been reported to have antioxidant properties that protect the body from free radicals (Hsu, Chen, Li, Chuang & Liu, 2006).

A breakthrough drug called recombinant human activated protein C (drotrecogin alfa, activated), or Xygris has emerged as the only drug with proven efficacy in treating life-threatening severe sepsis. It was approved by the U.S. Food and Drug Administration in November, 2001, and has a proven 29% relative risk reduction in patients at a higher risk of death. Activated protein C keeps coagulation in check and enhances fibrinolysis. Specific mechanisms for its clinical effect are not known, with more hurdles to overcome in the understanding of sepsis and its treatment (Eli Lilly and Company, 2010).

Randomized placebo-controlled studies have been done to examine the efficacy and safety of activated protein C. They concluded that treatment with drotrecogin alfa activated, significantly reduces mortality in patients with severe sepsis and may be associated with an increased risk of bleeding (Bernard et al., 2001).

It is important to note that sepsis starts with an infection, but antibiotics do not treat the out-of-balance immune response which produces excessive inflammation, coagulation, and impaired fibrinolysis which impairs blood flow and damages tissue and organs. Questions continue about the role of pro-tein C therapy in patients with severe sepsis, and additional trials are being conducted to identify appropriate candidates for treatment, and consensus concerning guidelines with sepsis (Toussant & Gerlach, 2009).

Solutions for early and accurate diagnosis of sepsis are evolving. A new DNA test for sepsis-causing bacteria called the Prove-it assay has resulted in the highly accurate and rapid detection of most common causes of sepsis (Peters, Savelkoul & Vandenbroucke-Grauls, 2010). The gold stan-dard for species identification is blood culture which can take one to three days to become positive, and another one to two days to identify the bacteria. The Prove-it test is fast and accurate and delivered results an average of 18 hours before conventional culture methods did, identifying sepsis-causing bacteria from a positive blood culture in only three hours, offering a major advance in the future diagnosis of sepsis (Mobidiag Ltd., 2010).

The SIRS-Lab in Jena, Germany has developed a molecular diagnostic test for sepsis called VYOO. Within 8 hours,

VYOO detects 99% of all sepsis-relevant bacteria and fungi as well as important resistances. VYOO allows better and faster therapy decisions than current standard procedures. Clinicians will be able to determine the most effective anti-infective therapy, benefiting the patient, as well as reducing overall costs and treatment times. Earlier diagnostics and rapid, accurate treatment can help reduce the sepsis mortality rate (SIRS-Lab, 2007).

Seegene Inc. is a molecular diagnostic company that has developed a Magicplex Sepsis Test, a new multi-pathogen test capable of quick and accurate identification of over 90 leading sepsis-causing pathogens. Their real-time PCR (polymerase chain reaction) method which provides results within three hours, quickly and comprehensively determines the levels of suspected targets in a patient's blood sample, and identifies drug resistant genes to better inform a diagnosis. Polymerase chain reaction is a method using an enzyme called polymerase to analyze short sequences of DNA of a specific organism (Seegene Inc., 2010). This test may become the new gold standard for performing accurate, rapid, and cost-effective sepsis diagnosis, answering the challenge to determine correct treatment of sepsis within the first few hours of the onset of the disease (Clinical Lab Products, 2010).

BioMerieux clinical diagnostics offers several solutions for diagnosing sepsis, including automated blood culture systems, identification and susceptibility systems, and automated tests for early diagnosis of sepsis and bacterial infection. Their VIDAS B-R-A-H-M-S PCT assay uses Procalcitonin (PCT) as a useful piece of the sepsis puzzle.

Procalcitonin is an early biomarker which is specifically increased during bacterial infection and sepsis, and is now recognized as a useful tool in the diagnostic process, helping with accurate, early, and differential diagnosis of infection/sepsis. The test to detect Procalcitonin takes just 20 minutes, making it possible to obtain early indications so that a patient can be given proper treatment. This can contribute to optimizing antibiotic therapy and monitoring treatment (Biomerieux, Inc., 2010).

The immune inflammatory response in the sepsis progression leads to immunosuppression and the immune system fails to eradicate the infectious pathogens. The immunotherapy approach for sepsis develops trials of immunostimulatory agents that may bring about a reversal of immunosuppression in sepsis. By studying the molecular mechanisms that underlie immune suppression following sustained inflammation, a major advance in sepsis treatment may be produced (Hotchkiss & Opal, 2010).

Another direction for understanding the character and process of sepsis is the development of educational materials that can contribute to early identification and treatment. Courses, videos, and tutorials can be found on the internet. One example is a one-hour online course for clinicians called: "The Early Identification and Management of Septicemia in the Acute Care Setting." This course was designed to meet the educational needs of critical care and infectious disease clinicians, and other health care providers involved in the care of patients with sepsis syndromes (Maves, 2010).

The Emergency Medicine Resident's Association has produced a handy pocket reference guide or EMRA Sepsis Card which is endorsed by the Surviving Sepsis Campaign. It is a compact, comprehensive review of the most recent recommendations for treating sepsis (Emergency Medicine Residents' Association, 2009).

I would anticipate the requirement of an entire course focused on sepsis in the medical college curriculum in the near future, which would cover all the basics about sepsis from the onset to the interventions and guidelines implemented by hospital staff. They might also include a post-discharge hospital rehab program guideline for recovery, designed specifically for sepsis survivors and their individual impairments. There is also a need for general brochures about sepsis, written in ordinary language, on the shelves in doctor's offices and other healthcare facilities, to help increase awareness about the under-recognized condition of sepsis.

After all the research so far, have the studies been successful at the implementation level in hospitals? The answer is, "yes." This is one example.

On August 30, 2010, Catholic Healthcare West (CHW), the nation's eighth largest health system announced that its severe sepsis prevention initiative has saved an additional 991 lives and reduced severe sepsis inpatient mortality by 33% at the end of three years. Using the Surviving Sepsis Campaign recommendations, as well as the Institute for Health Care Improvement's collaborative improvement methods, CHW caregivers and staff produced ground breaking work diagnosing sepsis earlier, treating it more aggressively, and saving lives (Catholic Healthcare West, 2010).

Although sepsis is running rampant, producing high mortality rates and devastating aftermaths, there is hope on the horizon. I want to end this chapter with HOPE, that continued dedication and commitment to research and treatment, combined with generous funding, will bring about great advances in sepsis which can save lives and help to heal people all over the world. Without knowledge, we perish.

CHAPTER NINE

REFLECTIONS

Give me beauty in the inward soul, may the outward and
the inward man be at one - Socrates

Looking somewhat perplexed, after staring at my intense
drawings and discussing my dark journey through the ICU
with severe sepsis, Dr. Micchia once asked me, "Is there any
Heaven at the other end?" Yes, there is, but I had to travel to
the edge of death, and struggle several times through a Purgatory-like realm of darkness to get there. My survival of
sepsis became a powerful, penetrating, life-changing event,
where my suffering and confinement eventually led me to a
greater liberation of my spirit and soul, and a richer life.

Severe sepsis was hell. Its fury unleashed through my body
like a raging California wildfire. I felt like it was obliterating
me, and quickly grinding me down to nothing. I felt stripped
from the inside out, as if my soul was laid bare. The pain
consumed me and my body was devastated, and I waited for
death's relief.

While the surface battle with my septic condition raged on in
the ICU, a concurrent spiritual confrontation began within
me as I neared death. I had other vivid dreams, deliriums,
and paranoid episodes, but nothing compared to my indelible

near-death experience into the black Purgatory-like realm of darkness. Here I felt lost, lonely, and helpless, trapped in a quagmire of sad moaning souls in what seemed like a waiting place between heaven and hell. There were no burning flames, and there was no heavenly throne. Was I on the boundary between heaven and hell? This was a deep, dark place full of anguish and despair. People just sat there grieving. It was void of love, light, and peace, but I still felt alive and conscious, and anxious to escape it.

Some unexpected things began to happen to me. Each time I descended into the realm of darkness it felt more frightening and powerful, trying to hold me. Sometimes I would catch a glimpse of non-human figures with glaring evil faces, but each time, after groping for an undetermined amount of time, I found a light at a tiny window on a door and escaped back to what I would call a realm of luminosity, where there was a peaceful soft presence within my room in the ICU.

This light was a Divine presence, God leading me back to the live, conscious world. My sister called me three months after I returned home from the hospital, and told me about the "presence" she felt moving into my room and alongside my bed. I had felt it then, but said nothing to anyone about it. These travels back and forth from that dark void to the conscious, light-filled room transpired right at the time that the doctors told my wife to call in the family, and that if I did not improve in the next 24-48 hours she would lose me.

So, what exactly is the, "heaven at the other end", after all of the horrible battles subsided? Simply put, in death there is life. My degenerative condition helped to bring about a regeneration of my soul and spirit, an area I had been neglecting for some time while I felt unappreciative of life, and was angry, complaining, and depressed about many things. God's light, love, and presence lifted me and brought me back from the edge of death, out of darkness and into a richer more meaningful life. My near-death experience helped me to unload some baggage that had choked and burdened my spiritual life, reminding me of the heavy chain carried by Marley's ghost in A Christmas Carol by Charles Dickens.

That Divine light and presence guided me to a door out of Purgatory several times, brought a healing presence next to my bed in the ICU, and soothed my spirit with a luminosity that dispelled the darkness in my life, gave me a greater sense of purpose, and a more refined, sentient, spiritual path to walk. That Divine love and light lifted me higher, out of illness, and into a better place, that place where miracles and healing happen and my encapsulations began to fall aside, and my mind and spirit soared. My perceptions of life began to change, and I found more joy in living. I call that healing, peaceful, spiritual power, the realm of luminosity.

It is a moment, or a time when I surrendered everything and opened up to a state of being where love and peace permeated my soul. I was ready to move on to "the next place" and discard my earthly concerns as I followed the light, but I was given back the gift of life, and that divine energy has remained a part of every one of my days. I deeply appreciate my new energized life.

I vividly remember the events that transpired, and have illustrated them in my art journal. I can easily close my eyes and see it all again, and again, reminding me of where I have been, and how far I have come forth out of darkness. Believe me, that horrible dark void is there, but God's Divine love, light, and healing is too.

When I would return from that Purgatory-like void, my family would often be waiting. My wife, sons, sisters, and other family members held my hand and talked to me softly. Their encouraging words and prayers were a great comfort to me. Sometimes I only saw them as shadow figures with orange bodies and a blue mist all around the room, but I felt their love and support.

Sometimes my thoughts raced through my mind. "I'm never going to see my wife and family again," I said to myself in a muffled, tired voice. "I won't do another drawing or painting, and I won't play guitar and record my music." I was letting it all go, as my mind desperately grabbed at familiar images, but they could not be touched or grasped. It was like throwing out excess weight and baggage to save myself from sinking into the deep eddies of swirling death. I had to cling to life and the light in my spirit within, while everything else seemed to float off into oblivion. Once you have experienced this type of surrender, you recognize your own temporal and fragile existence. With my soul laid bare, my heart opened and my life changed.

Here are some of the changes:

1. A greater appreciation for the gift of life
2. Less fear of death, and feeling more prepared for the next place
3. Feeling better about being myself, self-acceptance
4. More love, compassion, kindness, and sensitivity toward others

5. Less attachment to material things
6. Better sense of destiny and purpose(including writing this book)
7. Greater spiritual awareness, embracing spiritual things, but not formal religion
8. Greater appreciation for family and friends
9. Praying for other people, even those I don't know
10. Crying more easily in various situations
11. More vivid and meaningful dreams
12. Knowing that love and the light transcend the mere material world
13. Meditate to a quiet place more easily
14. A realization that my near-death experience brought me to a spiritual awakening
15. Knowing that God is the light, love, and the peace that lifted me up
16. Finding spiritual balance in mind, spirit, and soul
17. Knowing that the dark void or Purgatory-like realm of darkness exists
18. Knowing that God also exists, with a Divine healing, transcending, peaceful presence
19. Love lifted me in my darkest hour
20. Miracles do happen
21. True riches are spiritual
22. A spiritual life has substance, sentience, and meaning

My survival of sepsis has been multi-dimensional with many triumphs over physical, mental, and spiritual challenges. My near-death experience left an indelible imprint upon my consciousness and gave me a spiritual makeover from the inside out. The revisions and renewal brought me into a greater sense of balance, feeling more love and peace than I ever did before. My rational mind was silenced to make way for spiritual awareness, rejuvenation, and a more sonorous life. I have been lifted up, but not in some unapproachable echelon, but rather a down to earth, genuine, more radiant inner state of life. My suffering opened the way to happiness, and helped me gain insight into deeper meaning and appreciation of life.

Every day after I get up, I lift my hands in the air and thank God for being alive. I celebrate every day. God gave me a miracle. There is heaven at the other end.

CHAPTER TEN

THE ART JOURNAL

Art is a means to enter, to play with, to dance with, to wrestle with anything that intrigues, delights, disturbs, or terrifies us - Pat B. Allen

My art work has been a subconscious servant that illuminates the pain, suffering, and emotional storms that my mind, body, and spirit endured during my survival and recovery of sepsis. It became part of my therapy, and revealed my true feelings, perceptions, and experiences. By reliving these episodes and events, I confronted my fears and anxieties, and began to lift the burden of illness from my soul. My art has been a means of expression, a way to solve problems and develop understanding, and a spiritual path that has helped me fulfill my life.

After slowly regaining my hand coordination in my first month at home, I began to do the drawings which cover a period from September, 2009 to January, 2011. Each drawing will have a title, and/or a brief comment or interpretation.

Here is a list, starting from my first drawing:

1. Demented nurses torturing me, and they liked it
2. Shadow figures of my family, all I could see

3. Too many strangers, paranoia and fear begin
4. Worried and depressed
5. Catheter agony, with crazed nurses
6. The cooling blanket, with male nurses helping me
7. Terrified of Sepsis, jaundice and pain increase
8. Drugged and Controlled, by the evil hospital staff, a conspiracy
9. Breaking Out of the ICU
10. Death Certificate, they were waiting for me to die
11. Terror from Sepsis, I was about to explode
12. Doctors discuss my case
13. Rehab with kind therapists
14. Trying My Best, with encouragement from therapists
15. Paranoia Takes Over, I trust no one
16. Extreme Fever, lying on the cooling blanket, can only see shadow figures
17. Time Distortion in the ICU, something is wrong with the clock!
18. My World is Crashing In (from all sides)
19. Trapped In The Dark Void, I wanted out
20. The Radiance and Love, my wife touches me
21. Finally on My Feet in rehab
22. Doctors tell me good news
23. Captured Again, demented nurses torture me in the basement of the hospital
24. Tearing Out the PICC Line to escape
25. Deeply Sad, worrying about my gallbladder condition and impending darkness
26. Breaking Apart while trapped in Purgatory
27. My wonderful care and support group: my family, doctors, and nurses
28. Studio in The Woods, with the eccentric, sickly singer

29. The Horror of Sepsis. I felt it obliterating me
30. Becoming Septic, high fever and distortion
31. The Prison of Affliction, your hell is your own
32. Love Lifted Me!
33. Desperate Escape, from the Purgatory-like realm of darkness full of anguished souls
34. Feeling more alive, I begin to return
35. Losing the Baggage, letting go of some things in my life
36. Going for a Walk, out of body experience walking down the hall, but above the floor
37. Amsterdam Warehouse, musicians and band equipment
38. Reflecting about my life
39. A more peaceful existence
40. My smile is returning
41. In and Out, of the dark void or Purgatory-like place
42. Recurrent Dreams ,of the void and souls trapped in it
43. I Can Never Forget
44. I am going through serious changes
45. Flashback again
46. Inner Light, a more vibrant life begins
47. Embracing the Light, column of flames that were not hot, felt like Divine light
48. Ethereal Escape, out of my body with my spirit walking down the hall
49. Divine presence in the ICU
50. Breaking Out of the ICU, getting paranoid, fearful, wanting to run away
51. Is That Outside? coming out after 14 days in the ICU
52. Sepsis Breakdown

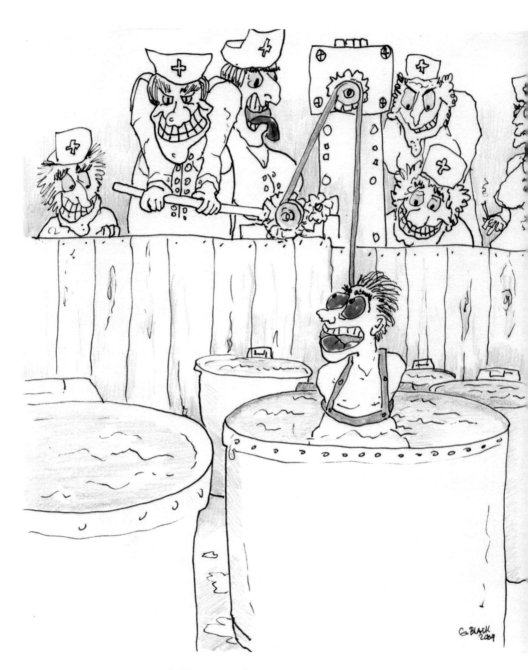

1. Demented Nurses Torturing Me

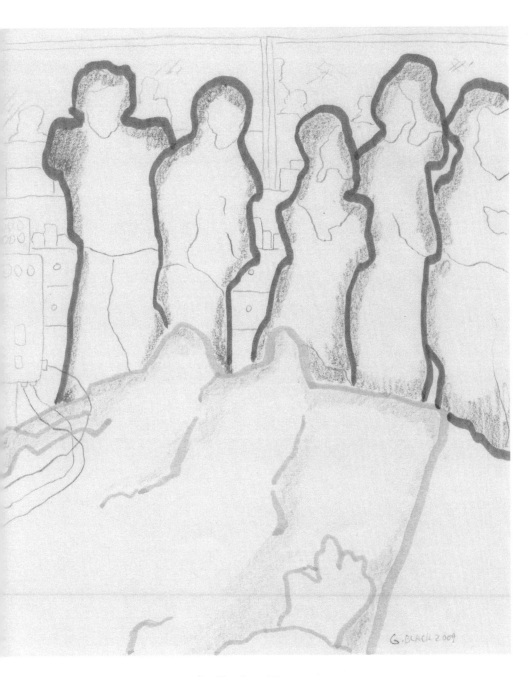

2. Shadow Figures

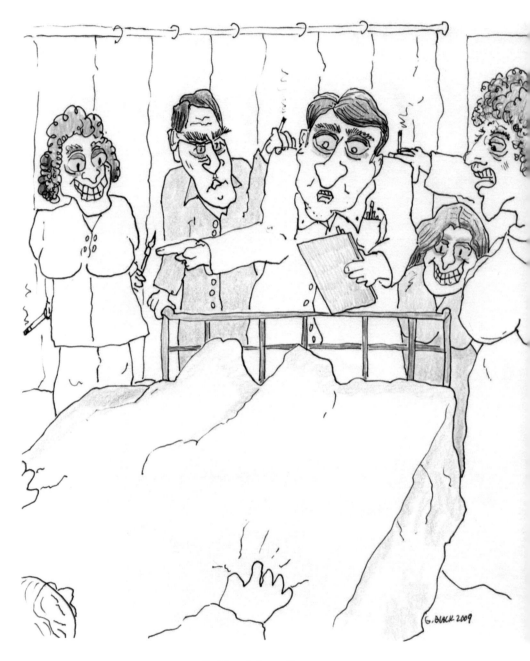

3. Too Many Strangers

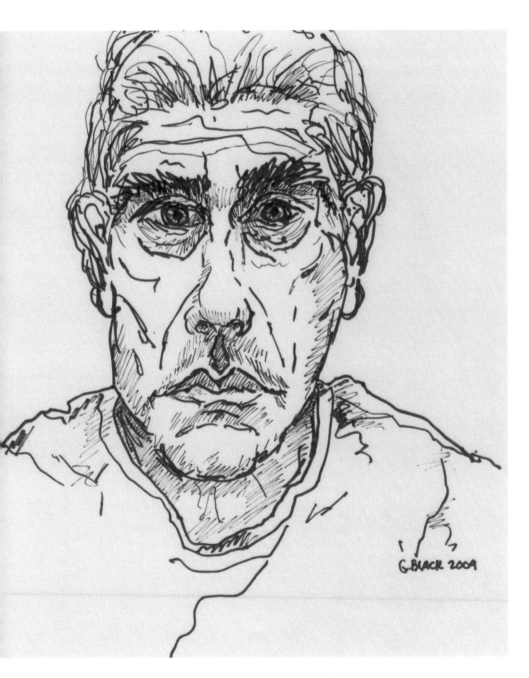

4. Worried and Depressed

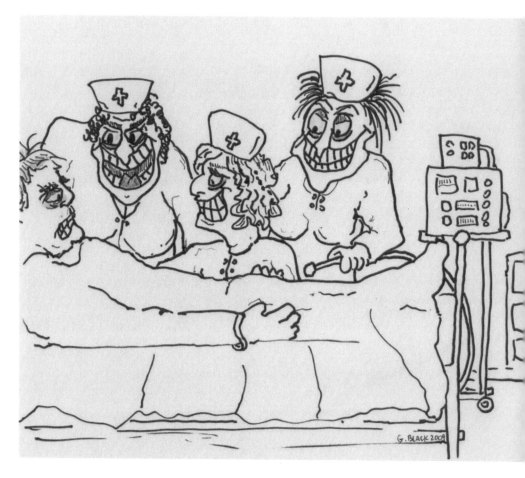

5. Catheter Agony

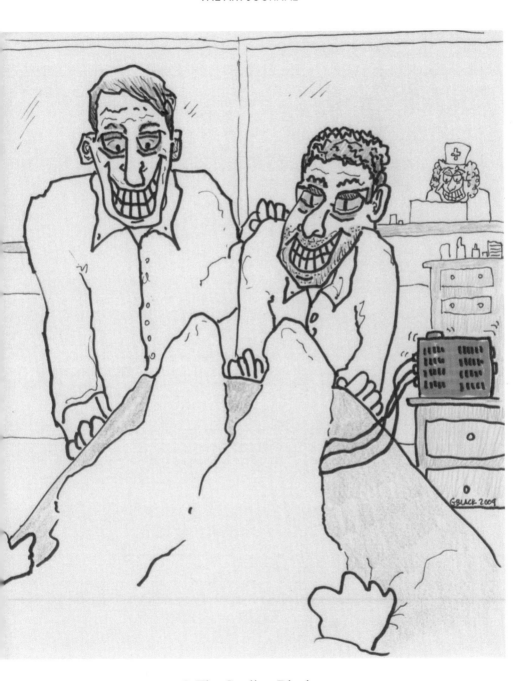

6. The Cooling Blanket

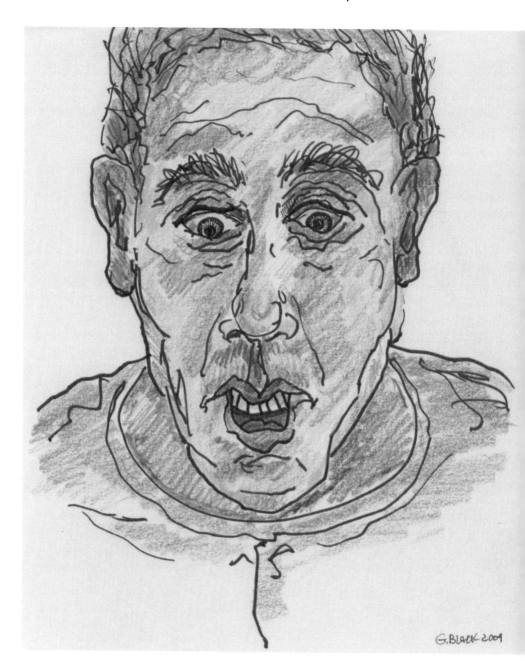

7. Terrified of Sepsis

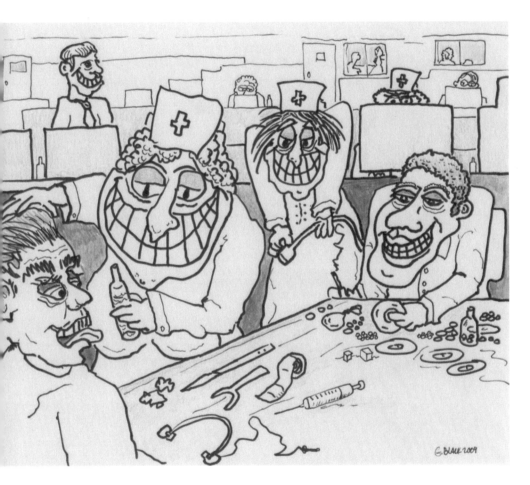

8. Drugged and Controlled

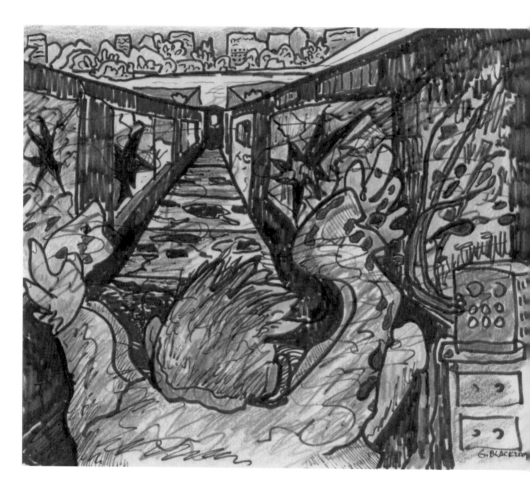

9. Breaking Out of the ICU

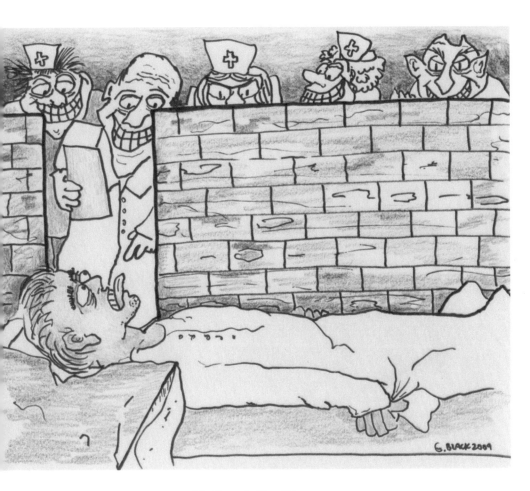

10. Death Certificate

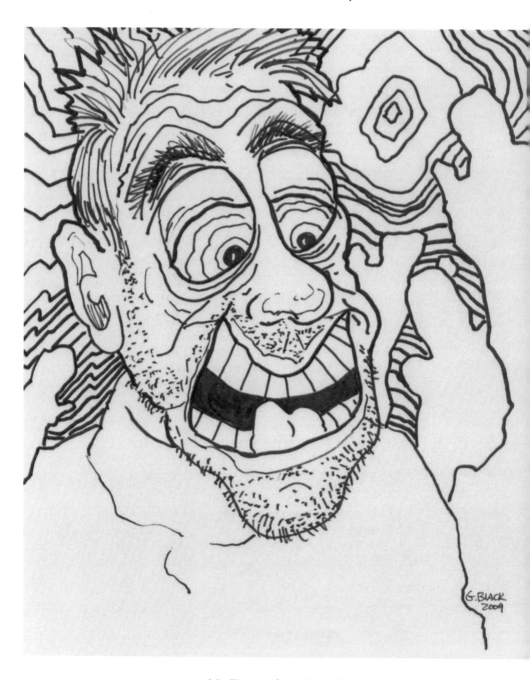

11. Terror from Sepsis

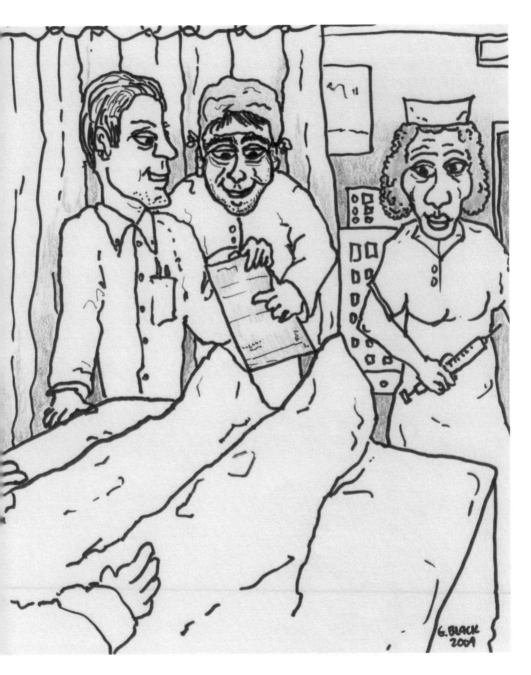

12. Doctors Discuss My Case

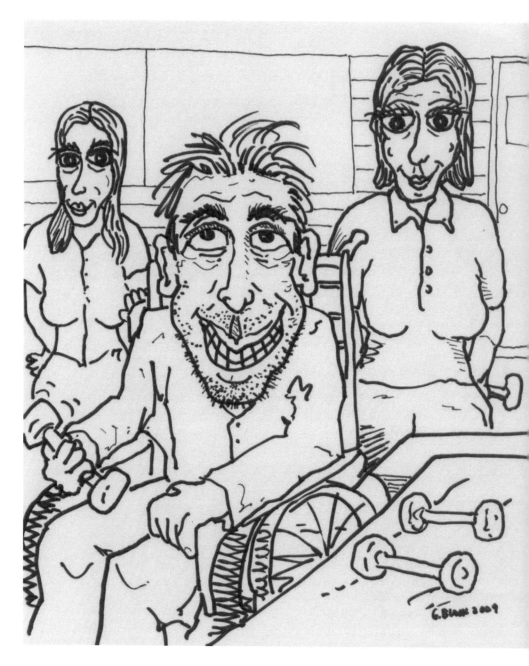

13. Rehab with Kind Therapists

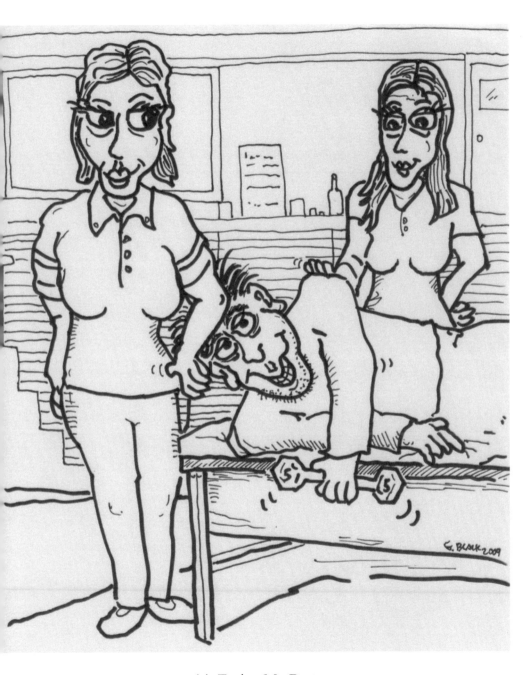

14. Trying My Best

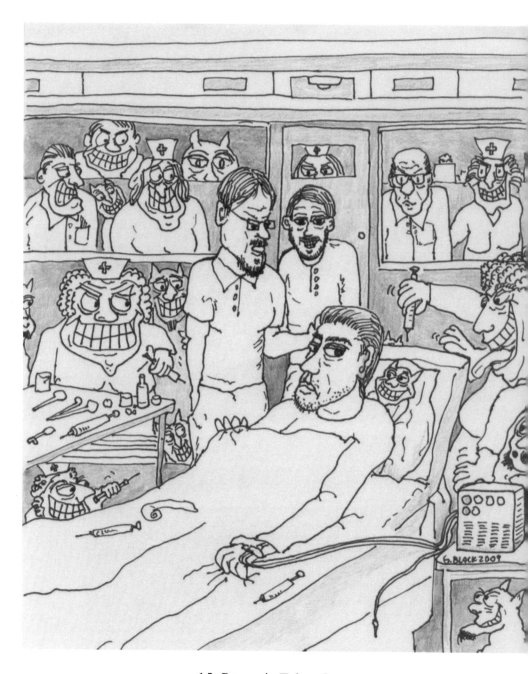

15. Paranoia Takes Over

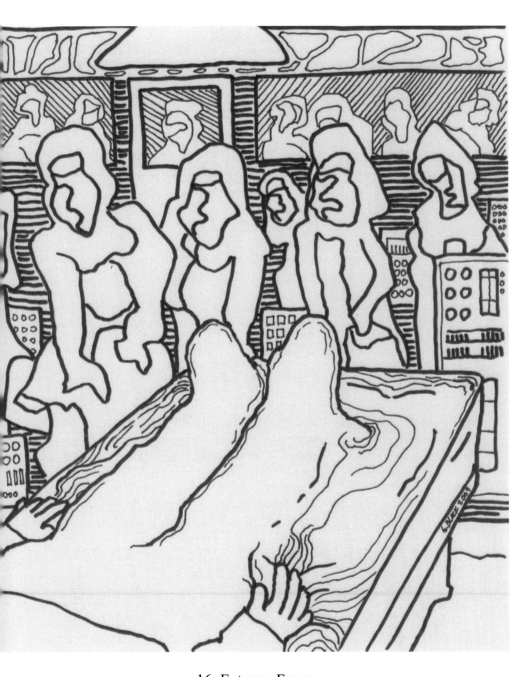

16. Extreme Fever

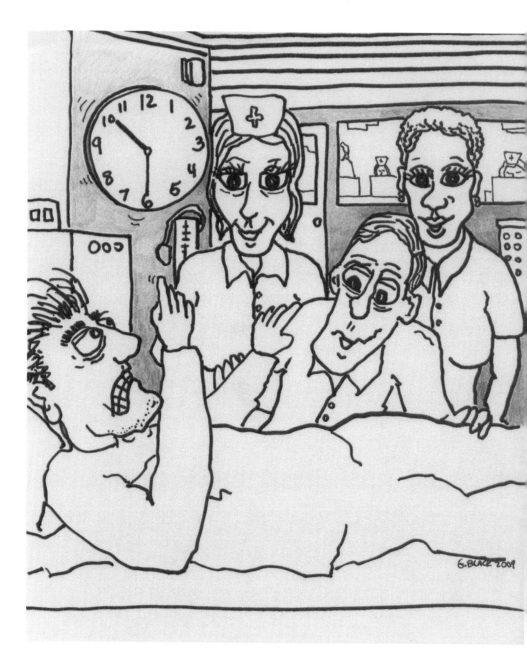

17. Time Distortion

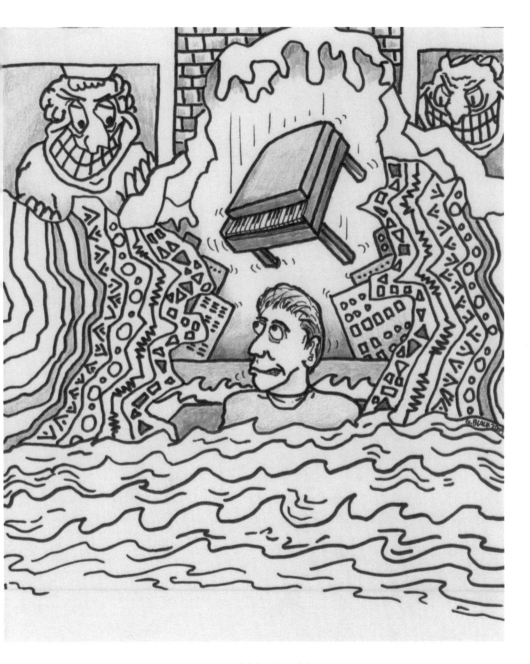

18. My World is Crashing In

the light of the window in the door

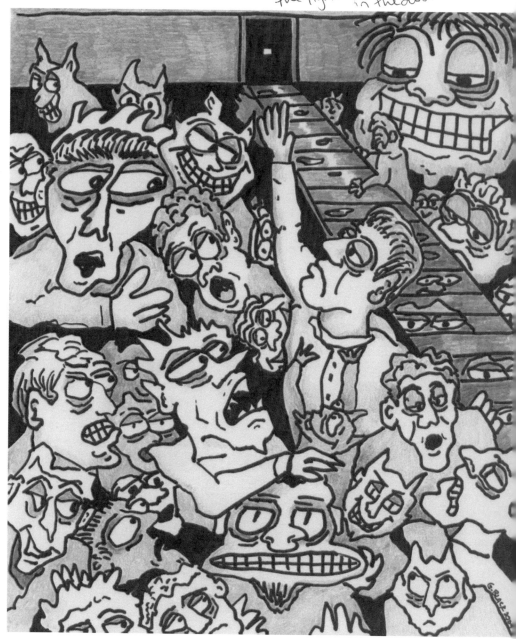

19. Trapped In The Dark Void

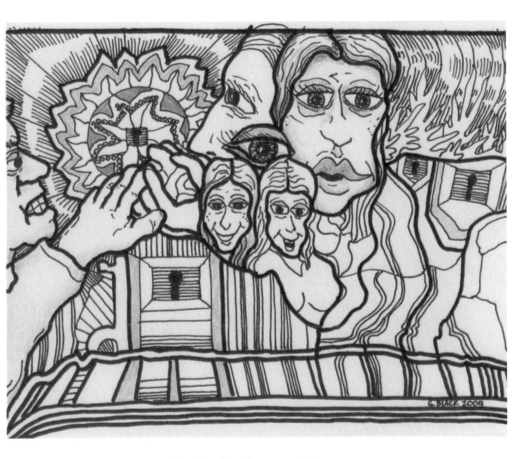

20. The Radiance and Love

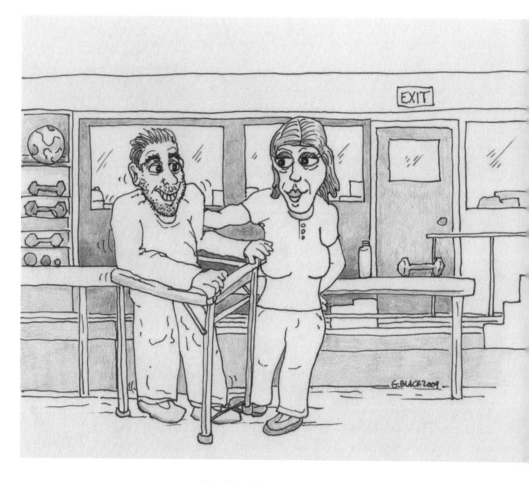

21. Finally on My Feet

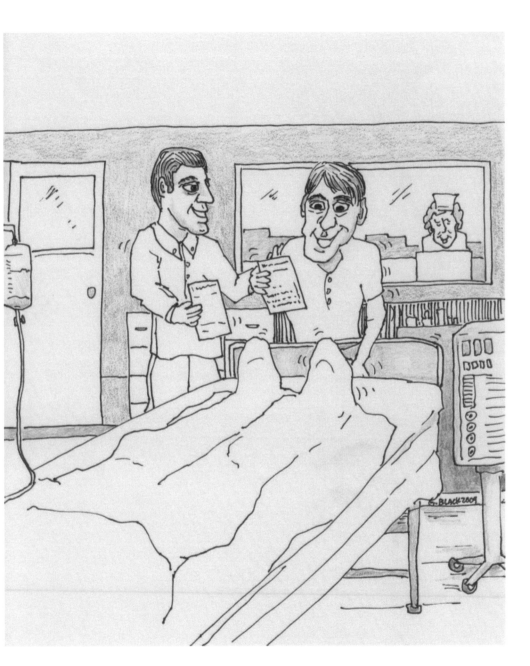

22. Doctors Tell Me Good News

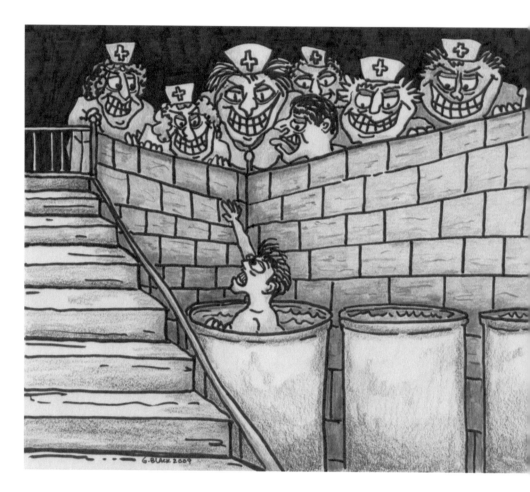

23. Captured Again

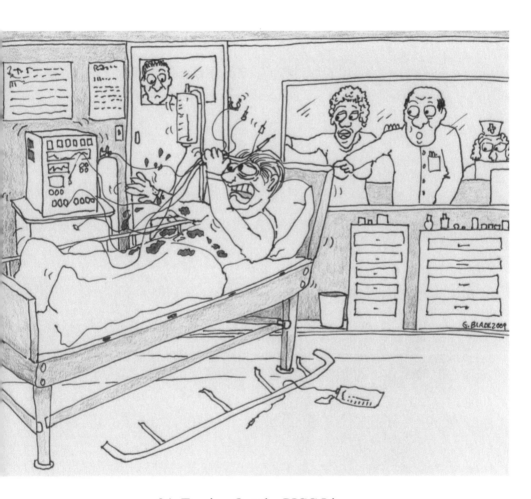

24. Tearing Out the PICC Line

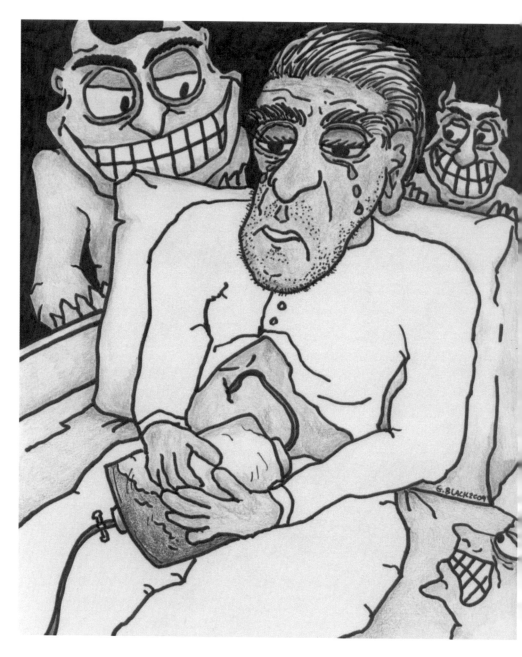

25. Deeply Sad

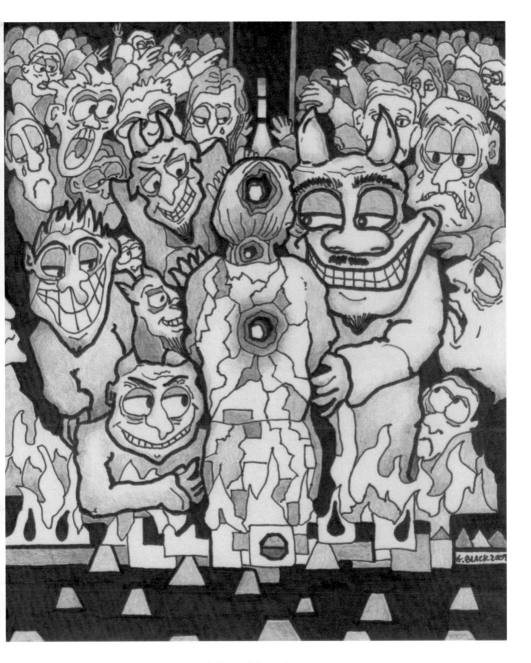

26. Breaking Apart

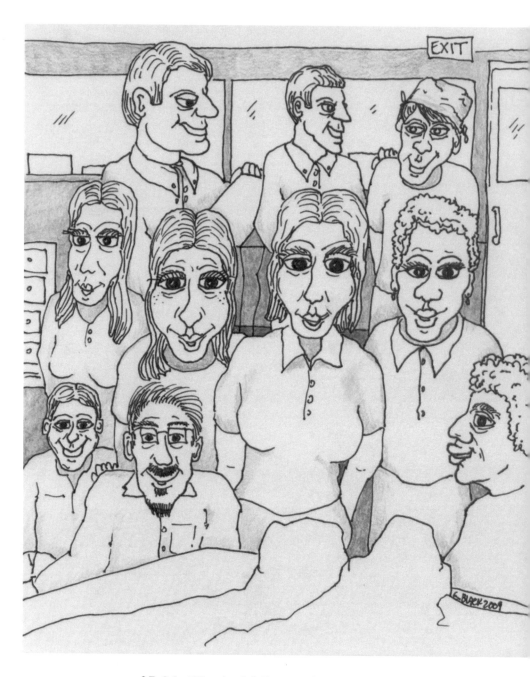

27. My Wonderful Care and Support Group

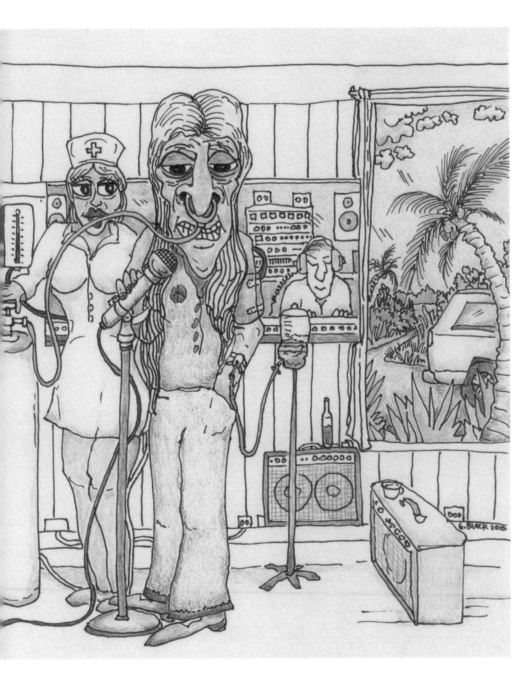

28. Studio in The Woods

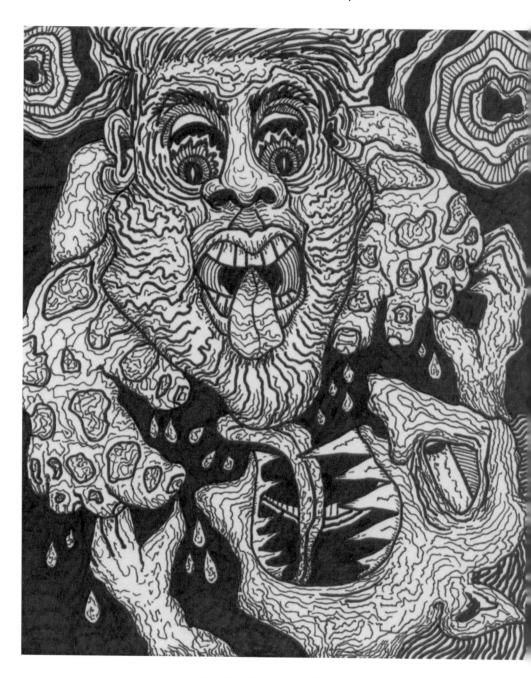

29. The Horror of Sepsis

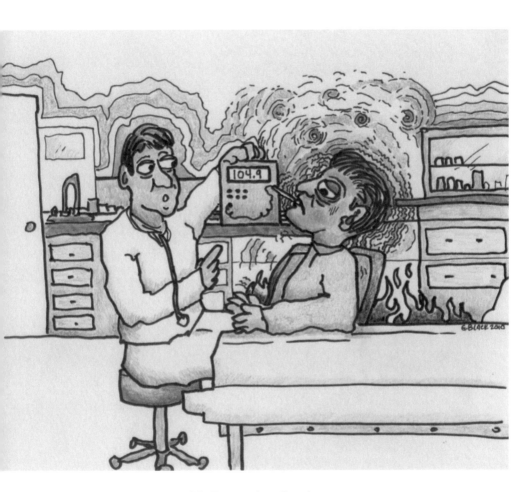

30. Becoming Septic

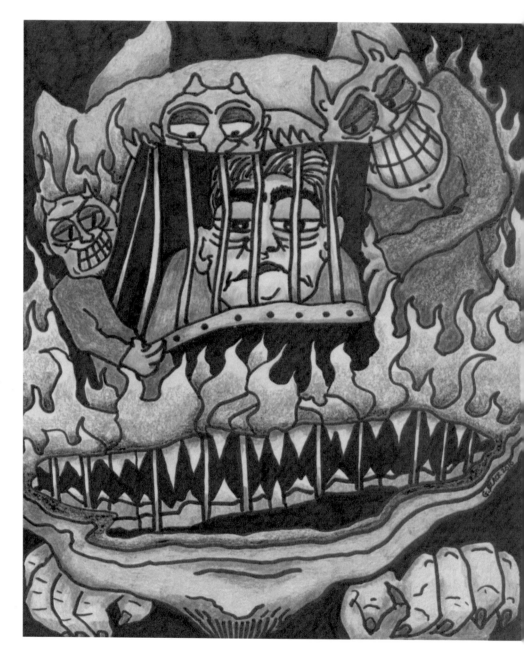

31. The Prison of Affliction

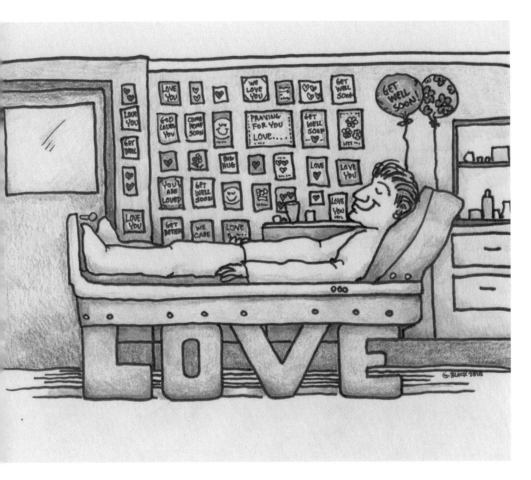

32. Love Lifted Me!

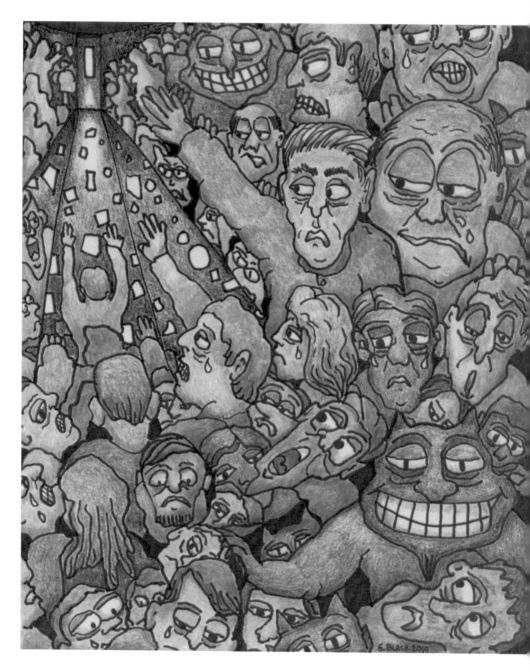

33. Desperate Escape

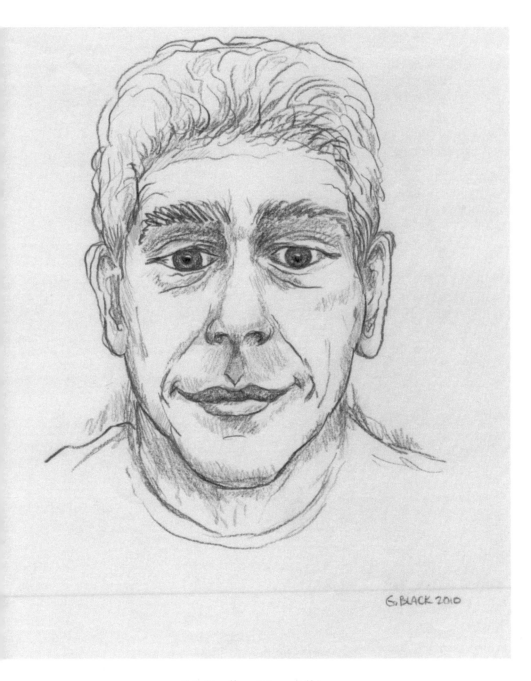

34. Feeling More Alive

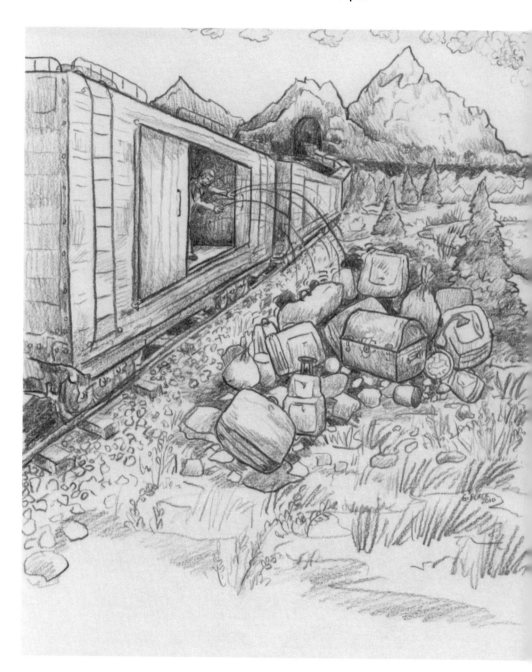

35. Losing the Baggage

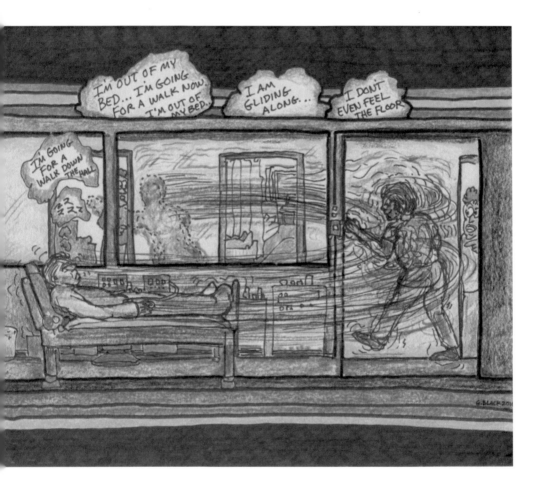

36. Going for a Walk

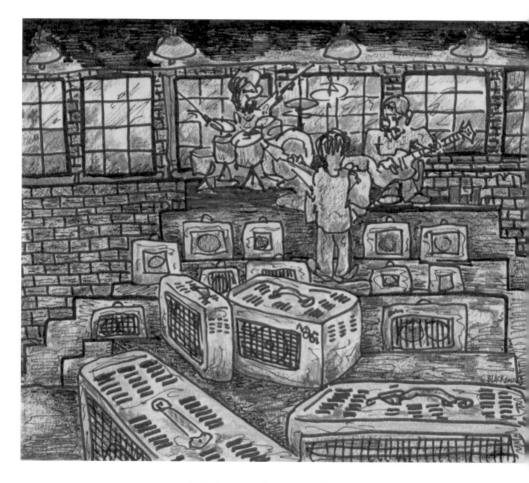

37. Amsterdam Warehouse

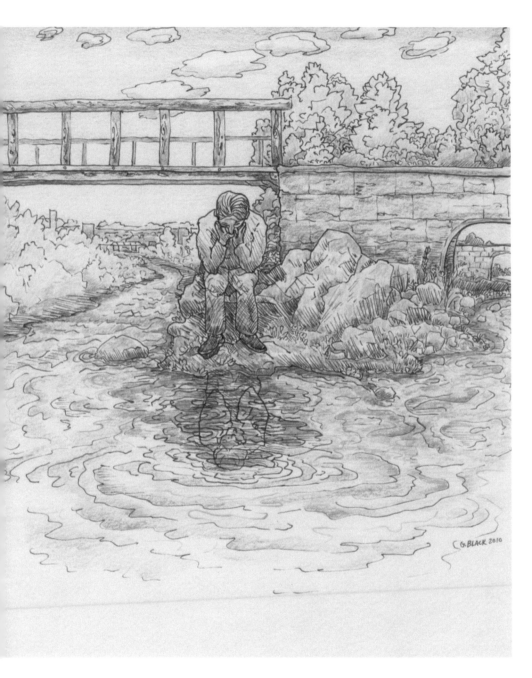

38. Reflecting About My Life

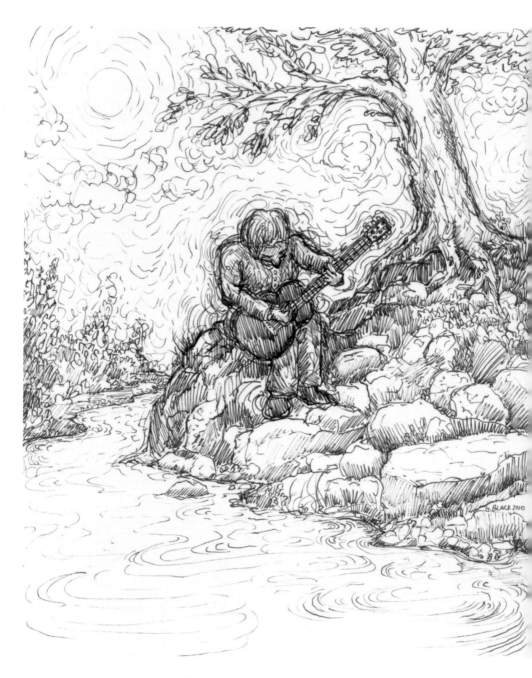

39. A More Peaceful Existence

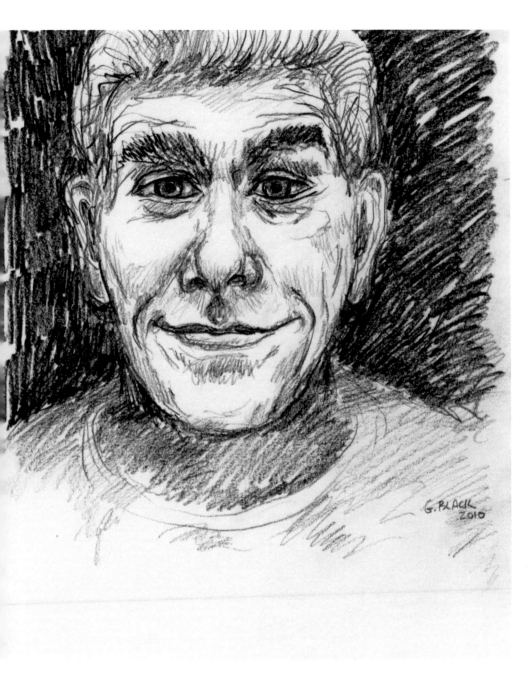

40. My Smile is Returning

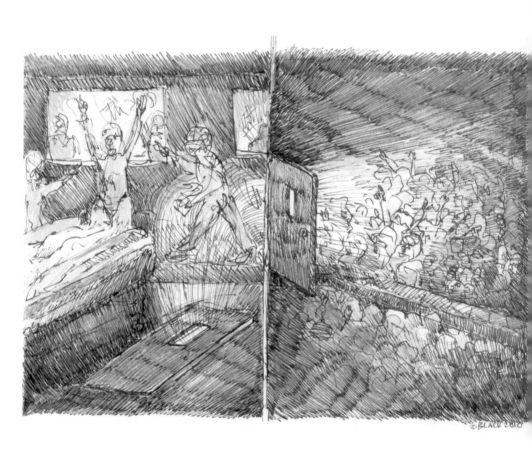

41. In and Out of the Dark Void

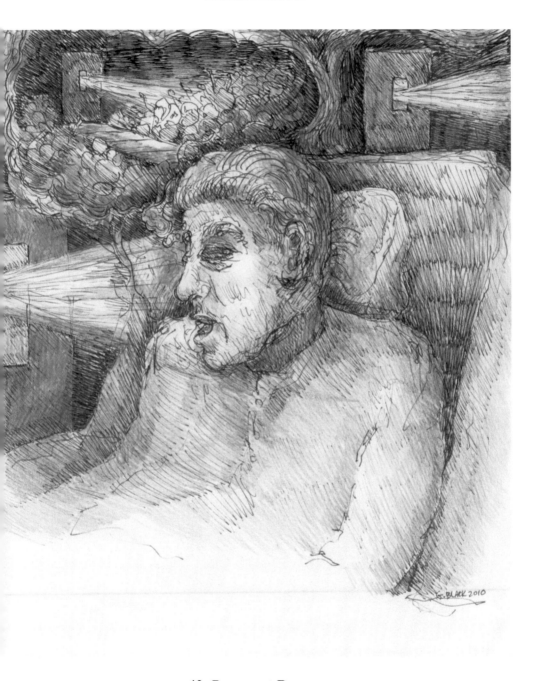

42. Recurrent Dreams

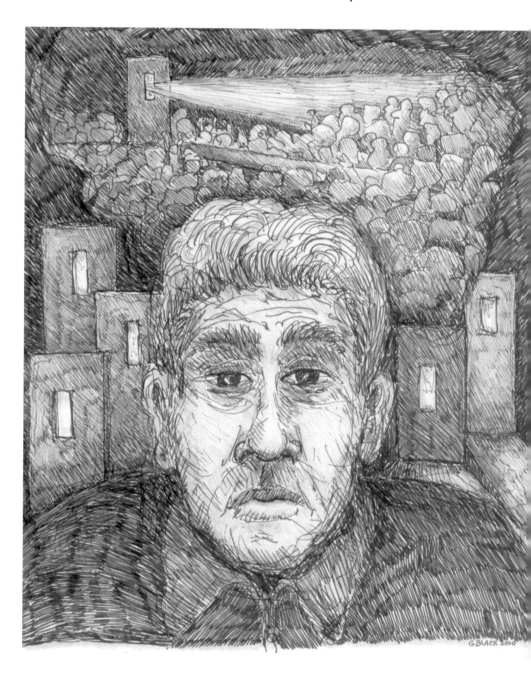

43. I Can Never Forget

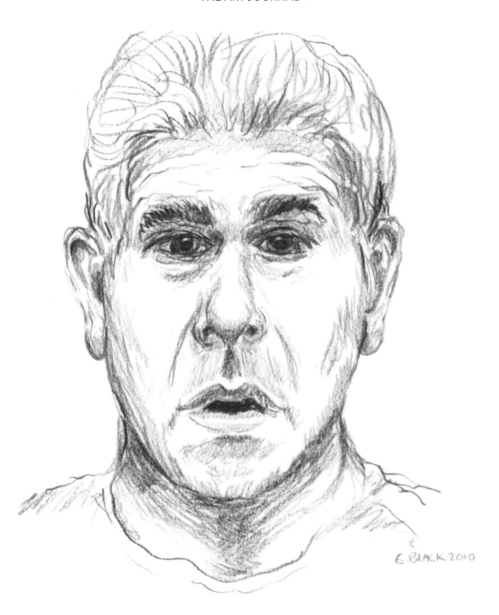

44. Serious Changes

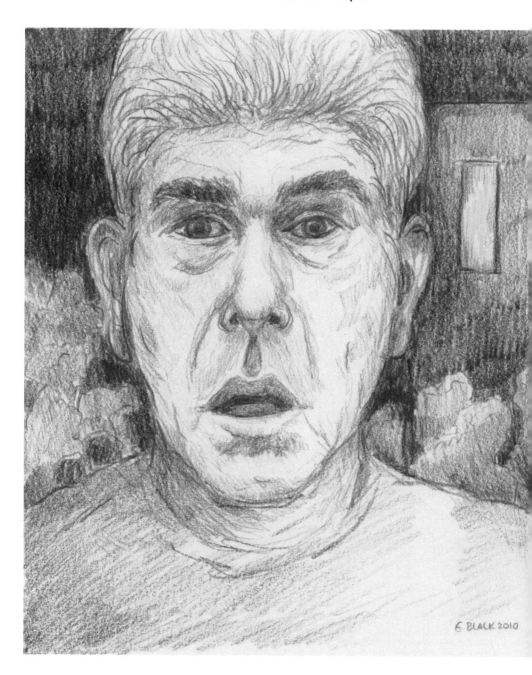

45. Flashback Again

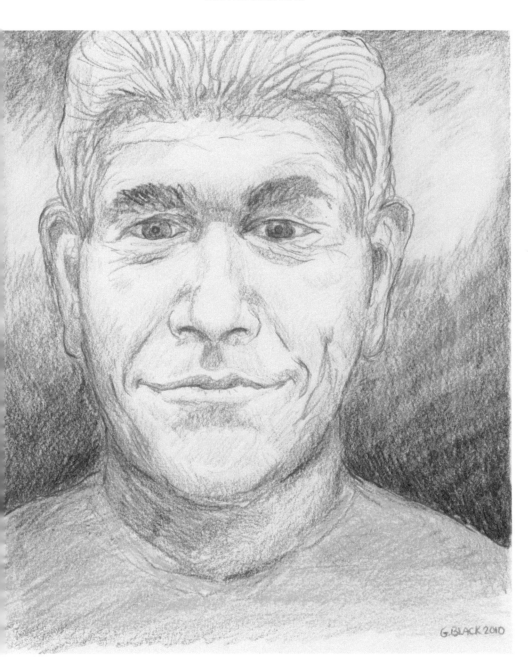

46. Inner Light

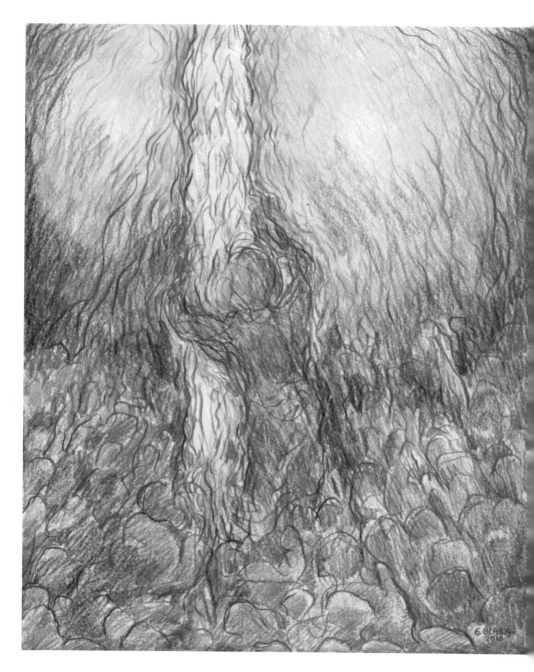

47. Embracing the Light

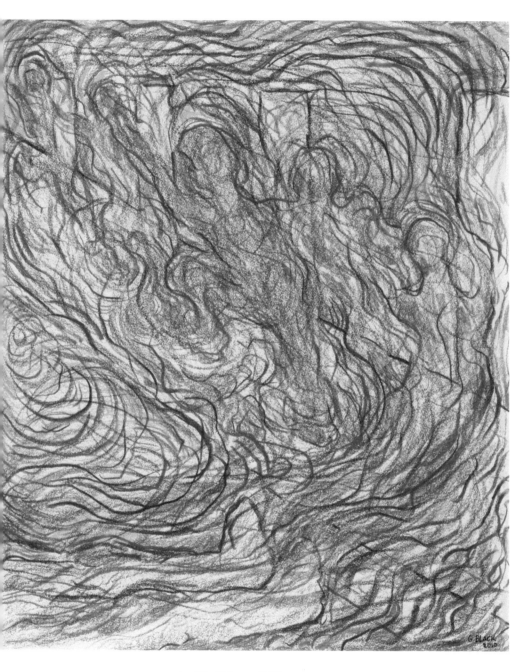

48. Ethereal Escape

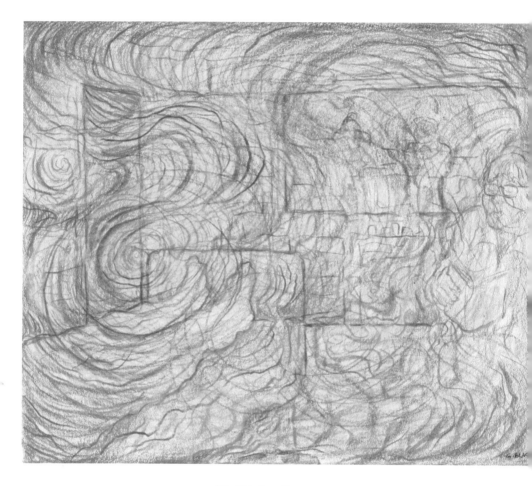

49. Divine Presence

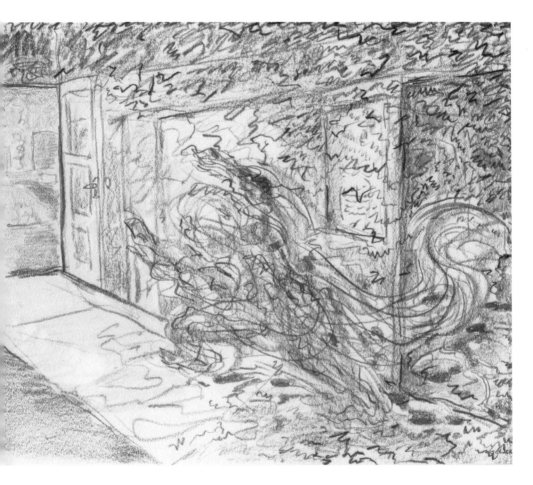

50. Breaking Out of the ICU

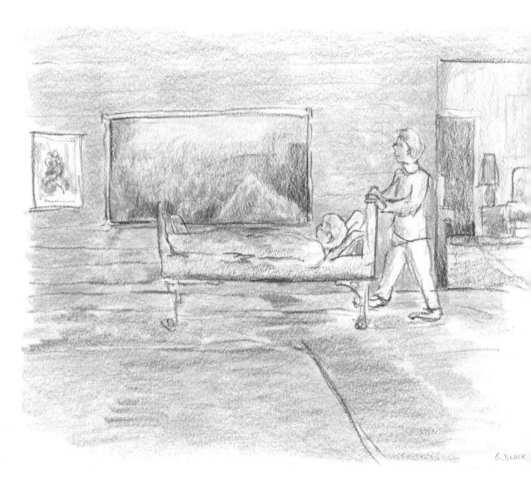

51. Is That Outside?

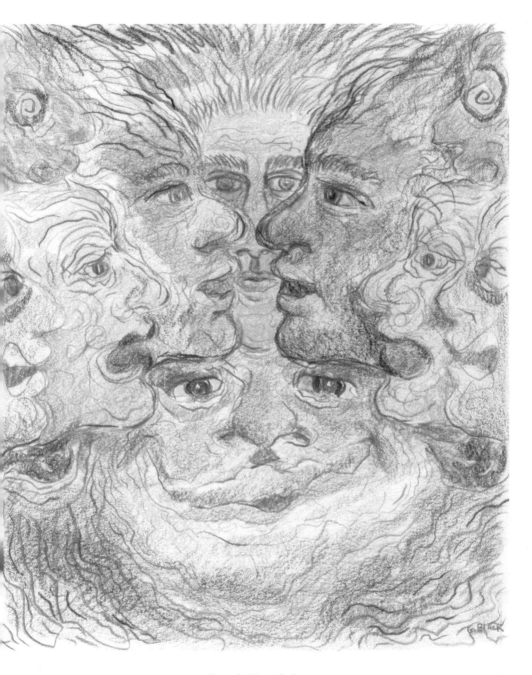

52. Sepsis Breakdown

GLOSSARY

Acalculous- Not effected with or caused by gallstones

Acetaminophen- Pain reliever, reduces fever

Albumin- Protein made by the liver

Anemia- Decrease in normal number of red blood cells, low oxygen transport capacity

Anesthesiologist- Doctors of Medicine (MDs) that concentrate on the care of surgical patients and pain relief

Anoxic- Oxygen deficient, absence or near absence of oxygen

Apnea- Suspended breathing, pauses in breathing, airway obstruction, decreased oxygen supply

Asymptomatic- Junctional rhythm, abnormal heart rhythm, no evidence of disease

Augmentin- Penicillin antibiotic used to treat infections

Biliary- Having to do with the gallbladder

Bilirubin- Yellow-colored pigment found in the bile, produced when the liver breaks down old blood cells

Biopsy- Test involving removal of cells for examination

Broad Spectrum Antibiotic- Antibiotic that treats a wide range of bacteria

Cholecystectomy- Surgical removal of the gallbladder

Cholecystitus- Inflammation of the gallbladder

Cholecystostomy- Surgical incision of the gallbladder using a tube to effect drainage of bile

Cholecystostomy tube- Drainage tube placed in gallbladder, through abdominal wall to drain bag

Coagulation- Complex process by which blood forms clots

Coagulopathy- Blood clotting problems, prolonged bleeding or not clotting normally

Colace- Stool softener to relieve constipation

Comorbidity- A disease or condition that coexists with a primary disease, existing simultaneously, but independently

Confabulations- Confusing imagination with memory and facts, narrative reports of events that never happened

CT Scan- Computerized tomography using data from multiple x-ray images, turning them into pictures on a screen

Delirium- Acute confusional state, rapid changes in brain function and mental states, consciousness, awareness, thinking, and emotions

Delusions- Unwavering belief in something untrue, irrational beliefs defying normal reasoning

Denervation- Loss of nerve supply

Dilaudid- semi-synthetic derivative of morphine

Doxycycline- Tetracycline antibiotic for treating infections

Dreams- Subjective experience of imaginary images, sounds, voices, thoughts, and sensations during sleep

Dulcolax- Laxative/softener to treat constipation

Edema- Swelling caused by fluid in body tissues

EKG- Electrocardiogram, a recording of the electrical activity of the heart

EMG- Electromyography, test used to record electrical activity of muscles, and detect abnormal electrical activity, intramuscular test uses a needle (serving as an electrode) inserted through the skin into the muscle, activity is shown on a monitor

Encephalopathic- State of altered brain function

Encephalopathy- Syndrome of global brain dysfunction, wide variety of disorders which can be caused by infection, organ failure, or intoxication

Epidemiology- Study of incidence, distribution, and control of disease in a population using representative samples and medical data

Famotidine- Inhibits stomach acid production

Fentanyl- Stronger pain killer for chronic pain, synthetic opiod more potent than morphine

Fibrinolysis- A process that occurs inside the body to break down clots

Folate- B vitamin which occurs naturally in foods, such as spinach or asparagus

Foley Catheter- Flexible tune inserted into the urethra of the bladder to drain urine

Gallbladder- Organ just below the liver, stores bile secreted by the liver

Gastroenterologist- A physician who specializes in the diagnosis and treatment of disorders of the gastrointestinal tract, including the stomach, small intestine, large intestine, pancreas, liver, gallbladder, and biliary system

Gastroenterology- Branch of medicine that studies the gastrointestinal tract and its diseases

Gram negative bacteria- Bacteria that do not retain the violet dye in gram staining, such as salmonella, E-coli

Gram positive bacteria- bacteria stained dark blue or violet by gram staining, such as streptococcus, staphylococcus, and bacillus

Grandiosity- Unrealistic sense of superiority or importance

Haldol- Haloperidol, strong tranquilizer and high potency antipsychotic used for treating psychotic states, false perceptions, delusions, delirium, agitation, and fear

Hallucinations- False or distorted sensory experiences that appear to be real perceptions

Hemoglobin- Protein in red blood cells that carries oxygen

Hepatic- Having to do with the liver

Hospitalist- Physician whose primary professional focus is the general medical care of hospitalized patients, specializes in inpatient care

Hypertension- Elevated blood pressure (high blood pressure)

Hyponatremia- Metabolic condition where there is not enough sodium (salt) in the body fluids outside the cells

Hypoxemia- Low level of oxygen in your blood

ICU- Intensive care unit, specialized ward for the care of critically ill patients

ICU psychosis- Changed mental state of a patient due to inherent environmental factors of the ICU, causing anxiety and restlessness

Immunosuppression- Suppression of the body's immune system and its ability to fight infections and other diseases

Inflammation- A response of tissue to injury caused by invading organisms, characterized by increased blood flow to tissue, causing increased temperature, redness, swelling, and pain recognized as a nonspecific immune response

IV- Intravenous access device such as a small tube or catheter

IV-NAC- Intravenous acetylcysteine used for acetaminophen overdose to reduce extent of liver injury

Jaundice- Yellowish staining of skin, mucous membranes, or eyes caused by high levels of bilirubin

Ketones- Compounds produced as by-products when fatty acids are broken down for energy in the liver and kidney

Lactic acidosis- low PH in body tissues and blood

Laparoscopic- Minimally invasive surgery, using small incisions, thin instruments, a video camera, and a monitor

Lethargic- Drowsy, sluggish, fatigued, apathetic, listless

Lovenox- Anticoagulant to reduce risk of deep vein thrombosis, reducing blood clots

Mononeuropathy- Damage to a single nerve or nerve group which results in loss of movement, sensation or other function

Morphine- Pain killer/opiate for severe and agonizing pain

Mortality rate- A measure of the number of deaths in a population

Motrin- Ibuprofen, non-steroidal anti-inflammatory drug used to relieve pain, swelling, stiffness

MRI- Magnetic Resonance Imaging, uses an enormous magnet and radio waves instead of x-rays to visualize detailed internal structures of the body

Multifactorial- Involving or depending on several factors or causes

Near-Death Experience (NDE)- An intense awareness, sense, or experience of "otherworldliness", whether pleasant or unpleasant, that happens to people who are at the edge of death

Necrosis- Death of living cells or tissues

Nephrolithiasis- Process of forming kidney stones

Nerve conduction study- Used to evaluate the function and ability of electrical conduction of motor and sensory nerves (nerve conduction velocity), surface EMG

Neuropsychologist- Doctor of Psychology who conducts evaluations to characterize behavioral and cognitive changes resulting from disease or injury

Nitrites- Byproduct of harmful bacteria, can be found in urine

Nosocomial- Hospital acquired infections

Occupational therapist- A health professional trained to help people who are ill or disabled to learn to manage their daily activities

Oliguria- Decreased or low output of urine

Oxycodone- Strong opiod analgesic medication used to relieve moderate to severe pain

Paranoia- A mental disorder characterized by systematized delusions, extreme irrational distrust of others, tendency to look for hidden meaning behind other people's actions

Pathogen- A disease producing agent such as a virus or bacteria

Pathophysiology- Study of the changes of normal mechanical, physical, and biochemical functions, either caused by disease or resulting from an abnormal syndrome

Physical therapist- A person trained and certified to design and implement physical therapy programs to help patients suffering from disease or injury, to improve mobility, relieve pain, and increase strength

PICC- Peripherally inserted central catheter, allows intravenous access for a prolonged period of time

Prilosec- Omeprazole, decreases stomach acid, treats gastroesophageal reflux disease (GERD), promotes healing of erosive esophagitis

Protonix- also used to treat GERD, decreases stomach acid

Psychosis- Psychotic disorder due to a medical condition, such as hallucinations or delusions with impaired reality and personality changes

Radiology- The branch of medicine that deals with the use of radioactive substances in diagnosis (X-ray, etc.), and treatment of disease

Red blood cells- Erythrocytes, principal means of delivering oxygen to the body tissues via the blood flow in the circulatory system

Reinnervation- Restoration of nerve function after it has been lost

Renal- Having to do with the kidney

Resuscitation- Reviving a person, restoring them to life

Rigors- Shaking, trembling during high fever

Rocephin- Broad spectrum antibiotic to fight bacteria

SCD- Sequential compression device, intermittent pneumatic compression system with inflatable sleeves (placed around lower leg), designed to limit deep vein thrombosis

Sepsis- Infection of the blood stream, whole-body inflammatory state

Sepsis Syndrome- Complex systemic inflammatory condition associated with infection

Septic shock- Sepsis induced hypotension and multiple organ dysfunction or failure

Severe sepsis- Sepsis with acute organ dysfunction, altered mental state, hypoxemia, oliguria, low platelets, inflammation, and coagulation

SIRS- Systemic Inflammatory Response Syndrome, inflammatory state affecting the whole body, frequently in response to infection

Speech pathologist- A therapist responsible for the evaluation and treatment of problems with speech and language

Syndrome- A set of signs and symptoms that tend to occur together which may reflect the presence of a particular disease or chance of developing a particular disease

Systemic- Affecting the entire body

Tachycardia- Rapid heart rate, exceeding normal rate, heart produces rapid electrical signals

Tachypnea- Abnormal rapid breathing

Tangential- Divergent or digressive, touching lightly

Thiamine- Vitamin B-1, helps body cells convert carbohydrates into energy

Thrombocytopenia- Presence of few platelets in blood (low platelet count), platelets help blood to clot

Toradol- Keterolac, non-steroidal anti-inflammatory drug, short-term treatment for moderate to severe pain

Ultrasound- High frequency sound waves are bounced off tissues to image internal body structures

Vancomycin- Antibiotic for treatment of bacterial infections

Venous Pooling- Accumulation of blood in the veins (of legs) due to gravitational pull when a person changes position from lying down to standing up, which may cause dizziness or fainting

Venous thrombosis- Blood clot that forms within a vein, can cause swelling and pain

Wilson's disease- Inherited disorder where there is too much copper in body tissue which can damage the liver and nervous system

White blood cell count- Number of white blood cells in the blood, used to determine the presence of infection

White blood cells- Leukocytes, cells of the immune system involved in defending the body against infections

Xigris- Drotrecogin alfa, a recombinant version of naturally occurring activated protein C, indicated for the reduction of mortality in adult patients with severe sepsis who have a high risk of death

Zosyn- Piperacillin/tazobactum, injectionable anti-bacterial combination designed to reduce the development of bacteria, combines an antibiotic with an enzyme inhibitor for efficacy

REFERENCES

Ahrens, T. (2007). Sepsis: Stopping an Insidious Killer. American Nurse Today, 2, 1-3.

Angus, D.C., Linde-Zwirble, W.T., Lidicker, J.,Clermont, G., Carcillo, J. & Pinsky, M.R. (2001) Epidemiology of severe sepsis in the United states: analysis of incidence, outcome, and associated costs of care. Critical Care Medicine, 29, 1303-1310.

Autism Speaks. (2010). Epidemiology Information Packet: Frequently asked questions. Retrieved January 23, 2010 from http://www.kintera.org/atf/cf/(2DB64348-B833-4322-837C-8DD9E6DF1SEE)Brochure_Epidemiology FAQ.pdf

Benjamin, C.F., Hogaboam, C.M. & Kunkel, S.L. (2004). The chronic consequences of severe sepsis. Journal of Leukocyte Biology, 75, 408-412

Bernard, G.R., Vincent, J. L., Laterre, P.F., LaRosa, S.P., Dhainaut, J.F., Lopez-Rodriguez, A., Steingrub, J.S.Garber, G.E., Helterbrand, J.D., Ely, E.W. & Fisher Jr., C.J. (2001). Efficacy and Safety of Recombinant Human Activated Protein C for Severe Sepsis. New England Journal of Medicine, 344, 699-709.

BioMerieux Inc. (2010). Solutions for Sepsis Diagnostics. Retrieved December 6, 2010, from http://www.Sepsis knowfromday1.com/sepsis-diagnostics.php.

Bone, R.C., Balk, R.A., Cerra, F.B., Dellinger, R.P., Fein, A.M., Knaus, W.A., Schein, R.M., & Sibbald, W.J. (1992). Definitions for sepsis and organ failure and guidelines for the use of innovative therapies In sepsis. The ACCP/SCCM Consensus Conference Committee.

American College of Chest Physicians/Society of Critical Care Medicine. Chest, 101, 1644-1655. doi : 10.1378/chest.101.6.1644

Bookofjoe. (2004). Why did Christopher Reeve die? Retrieved February 5, 2010 from http://blogcritics.org/ culture/article/why-did-christopher-reeve-die/page-2/

Brun-Buisson, C., Meshaka, P., Pinton, P. & Vallet, B.; EPISEPSIS Study Group. (2004). EPISEPSIS: A reappraisal of the epidemiology and outcome of severe sepsis in French intensive care units. Intensive Care Medicine, 30, 527-529. Retrieved January 27, 2010 from http://www.ncbi.nlm.nih.gov/pubmed/14997295

Canadian Institute for Health Information. (2009) In Focus: A National Look at Sepsis. Ottawa, Ontario: CIHI. Retrieved January 29, 2010 from http://secure.cihi.ca/ cihiweb/products/HSMR Sepsis2009_e.pdf.

Carsten, L. (2010). MedaSorb optimistic to get EU approval for Blockbuster Product. Retrieved February 17, 2010 from http://endsepsis.org/blog/2010/02/04/medasorb-optimistic-to-get-eu

Castellanos-Ortega, A., Suberviola, B., Garcia-Astudillo, L.A., Holanda, M.S., Ortiz, F., Llorca, J. & Delgado-Rodriguez, M. (2010). Impact of the Surviving Sepsis

Campaign protocols on hospital length of stay and mortality in septic shock patients: results of a three-year follow-up quasi-experimental study. Critical Care Medicine, 38, 1036-1043.

Catholic Healthcare West. (2010). "Ground breaking" Severe Sepsis Prevention Program Saves 991 Lives, Reduces Costs by $36.5 Million. Retrieved October 20, 2010 from http://www.chwhealth.org/stellent/groups/public/@xinternet_con_sys/documents/webcontent/209932.pdf

Chang, H.J., Lynm, C., & Glass, R.M. (2010). Sepsis. Journal of the American Medical Association, 303,804

Chu, J. (2008). Microfiltering Sepsis. Retrieved February 17, 2010 from http://www.technologyreview.com/bio medicine/20816/

Cleveland Clinic. (2010). Diseases & Conditions, Sepsis Overview. Retrieved January 18, 2010 from http://my.clevelandclinic.org/disorders/sepsis/hic_sepsis.aspx

Clinical Lab Products. (2010). New Sepsis Test Identifies Over 90 Indicators for Deadly In-Hospital Disease. retrieved September 10, 2010 from http://www.clp mag.com/news/2010-07-26_02.asp

Comim, C.M., Constantino, L.C., Baricello, T., Streck, E.L., Quevedo, J. & Dal-Pizzol, F. (2009) Cognitive Impairment in the septic brain. Current Neurovascular Research, 6, 194-203 Epub 2009 Aug 1.

Decker, T. (2004). Sepsis: avoiding its deadly toll. Journal of Clinical Investigation,113, 1387-1389.

Dombrovskiy, V.Y., Martin, A.A., Sunderram, J., & Paz, H.L. (2007). Rapid increase in hospitalization and mortality rates for severe sepsis in the United States: a trend analysis from 1993 to 2003. Critical Care medicine, 35, 1244-1250.

Eli Lilly and Company. (2010). Sepsis: A Background Guide. Retrieved January 15, 2010 from http://www.lilly.com/pdf/sepsis_backgrounder_1003_vr3.pdf

Emergency Medicine Residents' Association (EMRA) (2009). EMRA Sepsis Card 2009 Edition. Retrieved August 20, 2010 from http://www.emra_bookstore.aspx?id=34264

Feinstein Institute for Medical Research. (2010). Most U.S. Adults Unfamiliar with Sepsis, One of Nation's Leading Causes of Death. http://www.northshorelij.com/NSLIJ/Most+US+Adults +Unfamiliar+with+sepsis.

Flatley, C.J., Sepsis Alliance. (2002). In Memory of Erin "Bug" Flatley, 1979-2002. Retrieved February 8, 2010 from http://www.sepsisalliance.org/about/erin/

German Sepsis Society. (2010). Aims and Objectives. Retrieved August 20, 2010 from http://www.sepsis.gesellschaft.de/DSG/Englisch

Global Sepsis Alliance. (2010). GSA Objectives. Retrieved August 20, 2010 from http://www.globalsepsisalliance.org/

Global Sepsis Alliance. (2010). Merinoff Symposium. Retrieved December 3, 2010 from http://www.global sepsisalliance.org/about/

Herr, H.W. (2007). Ignorance is Bliss: The Listerian Revolution and Education of American Surgeons. Journal of Urology, 177, 457-460. doi : 10.1016/j.juro.2006.09.066

Hofhuis, J.G.M., Spronk, P.E., van Stel, H.F., Schrijvers, A.J.P., Rommes, J.H. & Bakker, J. (2008). The Impact of Severe Sepsis on Health-Related Quality of Life: A Long-Term Follow-Up Study. Anesthesia & Analgesia, 107, 1957-1964.

Hopper, K. (2009). Halting the Sepsis Cascade. Cerner Quarterly, 5, 15-18.

Hotchkiss, R.S. & Opal, S. (2010). Immunotherapy for Sepsis-A New Approach against an Ancient Foe.New England Journal of Medicine, 363, 87-89

Hsu, D.Z., Chen, K.T., Li, Y.H., Chuang, Y.C. & Liu, M.Y. (2006). Sesamol Delays Mortality and Attenuates Hepatic Injury After Cecal Ligation and Puncture in Rats: Role of Oxidative Stress. Shock, 25, 528-532. doi : 10.1097/01.shk.0000209552.95839.43

International Sepsis Forum. (2010). Improving Sepsis Outcomes. Retrieved August 16, 2010 from http:// www.sepsisforum.org/

Iwashyna, T.J., Ely, E.W., Smith, D.M., & Langa, K.M. (2010). Long-term Cognitive Impairment and Functional Disability Among Survivors of Severe Sepsis. Journal of

the American Medical Association, 304, 1787-1794. doi
: 10.1001/jama.2010.1553

Jaimes, F. (2005). A literature review of the epidemiology of
sepsis in Latin America. Revista Panamericana de Salud
Publica, 18, 163-171. Retrieved January 27, 2010 from
http://www.scielosp.org/pdf/rpsp/v18n3/27665.pdf

Jones, C., & Griffiths, R.D. (2006). Long-Term Care of
Patients After Discharge from the Intensive Care Unit.
Advances in Sepsis, 5, 88-93

Karlsson, S., Ruokonen, E., Varpula, T., Ala-Kokko, T.I., &
Pettila, V. for the Finnsepsis Study Group. (2009).
Long-term outcome and quality-adjusted life years after
severe sepsis. Critical Care Medicine, 37, 1268-1274.
doi : 10.1097/CCM.0b013e31819c13ac

Kleinpell, R. (2003). Advances in Treating Patients With
Severe Sepsis. Critical Care Nurse, 23, 16-29.

Kotcheff, T. (1982). First Blood. USA: Orion Pictures.

Lazosky, A., Young, G.B., Zirul, S., & Phillips, R. (2009).
Quality of life after septic illness. Journal of Critical
Care, November 13, 2009 (Epub ahead of print). Retrieved January 29, 2010 from http://www.ncbi.nlm.
nih.gov/pubmed/19914034.

Levy, M.M., Fink, M.P., Marshall, J.C., Abraham, E., An-
gus, D., Cook, D., Cohen, J., Opal, S.M., Vincent, J.L.,
& Ramsay, G. (2003). 2001
SCCM/ESICM/ACCP/ATS/SIS International Sepsis

Definitions Conference. Intensive Care Medicine, 29, 530-538. doi : 10.1007/s00134-003-1662-x.

Martin, G., Brunkhorst, F.M., Janes, J.M., Reinhart, K., Sundin, D.P., Garnett, K. & Beale, R. (2009).The international PROGRESS registry of patients with severe sepsis: drotrecogin alfa (activated) use and outcomes. Critical Care, 13, R103. doi : 10.1186/cc7936 Retrieved February 2, 2010 from http://www.ccforum.com/content/13/3/R103

Martin, G.S., Mannino, D.M., Eaton, S., & Moss, M. (2003). The Epidemiology of Sepsis in the United States from 1979 through 2000. New England Journal of Medicine, 348, 1546-1554.

Maves, M. (2010). Sepsis Prevention, tutorial. Retrieved February 5, 2010 from http://www.faculty.Alverno.edu/bownesp/new indexes/MSN621201index.html

Melamed, A., & Sorvillo, F.J. (2009). The burden of sepsis-associated mortality in the United States from 1999 to 2005: an analysis of multiple-cause-of-death data. Critical care, 13:R28 doi : 10.1186/cc7733

Merinoff Symposia. (2010). 2010: Sepsis Overview. Retrieved December 3, 2010 from http://www.merinoff symposia.com/index.

Mobidiag Ltd. (2010). Prove-it Sepsis., Rapid Molecular Diagnostics for Sepsis. Retrieved August 10, 2010 from http://www.mobidiag.com/LinkClick.aspx?fileticket=Li o8QmQz-9g%3d&tabid=60

Nelson, D.P., Lemaster, T.H., Plost, G.N., & Zahner, M.L. (2009). Recognizing Sepsis in the Adult Patient. American Journal of Nursing, 109, 40-45.

Novartis Diagnostics Global. (2010). Disease Education, Disease glossary. Retrieved January 21, 2010 from http://www.novartisdiagnostics.com/

Ohio State Sepsis Registry. (2009). Retrieved January 30, 2010 from http://www.clinicaltrials.gov/ct2/show/study/NCT00837421

Opal, S. (2007). A brief history of sepsis: Landmarks in the understanding of severe infection and sepsis. http://www.imresidents.mhri.org/classroom/Hx-sepsis.ppt

Padkin, A., Goldfrad, C., Brady, A.R., Young, D., Black, N., & Rowan, K. (2003). Epidemiology of severe Sepsis occurring in the first 24 hours in intensive care units in England, Wales, and Northern Ireland. Critical Care Medicine, 31, 2332-2338. doi : 10.1097/01.ccm.0000085141

Parker, M.M. (editor) (n.d.). Editorial, Surviving Sepsis. Retrieved February 11, 2010 from http://www.advances insepsis.com/details.aspx?itemid=2043

Peters, R.P.H., Savelkoul, P.H.M., & Vandenbroucke-Grauls, C.M.J.E. (2010). Future Diagnosis of Sepsis. The Lancet, 375 (9728), 1779-1780.

Pulmonary Reviews. (2001). The National Impact of Severe Sepsis. Pulmonary Reviews, 6, 10. Retrieved January

23, 2010 from http://www.pulmonaryreviews.com/
oct01/pr_oct01_sepsis.html

Quartin, A.A., Schein, R.M., Kett, D.H. & Peduzzi, P.N.
(1997). Magnitude and duration of the effect of sepsis
on survival. Department of Veterans Affairs Systemic
Sepsis Cooperative Studies Group. Journal of the American Medical Association, 277, 1058-1063. Retrieved
January 29, 2010 from http://www.ncbi.nlm.
nih.gov/pubmed/9091694

Rello, J. & Restreppo, M.I. (Eds.) (2008). Sepsis: New Strategies for Management (p. 104) Berlin Heidelberg:
Springer-Verlag.

Rublee, D., Opal, S.M., Schramm, W., Keinecke, H.O. &
Knaub, S. (2002). Quality of life effects of anti-thrombin
III in sepsis survivors: results from the KyberSept trial
(SRCTN22931023).Critical Care, 6, 349-356. Published
online 2002, June 24.

Rubulotta, F.M., Ramsay, G., Parker, M.M., Dellinger, R.P.,
Levy, M., & Poeze, M. (2009). An international survey:
Public awareness and perception of sepsis. Critical Care
Medicine, 37, 167-170.doi:10.1097/CCM.obo13e3181
926883

Seegene Inc. (2010). Magicplex, New Concept in Multiplex
Real-time PCR. Retrieved September 10, 2010 from
http://www.seegene.com/en/magic/magic.php

Sepsis Alliance. (2002). About Sepsis Alliance. Retrieved
August 16, 2010 from http://www.sepsisalliance.org/
about/

Shen, H.N., Lu, C.L. & Yang, H.H. (2010). Epidemiologic trend of severe sepsis in Taiwan from 1997 through 2006. Chest, 138, 298-304. Retrieved January 26, 2010 from http://chestjournal.chestpubs.org/content/138/2/298

SIRS-Lab. (2007). Molecular Diagnostics for Sepsis. Retrieved august 13, 2010 from http://www.sirs-lab.com/english/company/about-sirs-lab.html

Society of Critical Care Medicine. (2002).Surviving Sepsis Campaign, About the Campaign. Society of Critical Care Medicine, European Society of Critical Care Medicine & the International Sepsis Forum. Retrieved February 15, 2010 from http://www.survivingsepsis.org/ About_the_Campaign/Pages/default.aspx

Society of Critical Care medicine. (2002). Surviving Sepsis Campaign: Action demanded on World's oldest killer. Retrieved October 10, 2010 from http://www.survivngsepsis.org/Background/Pages/world 'soldestkiller.aspx

Sundararajan, V., Macisaac, C.M., Presneill, J.J., Cade, J.F. & Visvanathan, K. (2005). Epidemiology of Sepsis in Victoria, Australia. Critical Care Medicine, 33, 71-80. Retrieved January 29, 2010 from http://www.ncbi.nlm. nih.gov/pubmed/15644651

Thompson, J. (2005). Making a difference out of her memory. St. Petersburg Times. Retrieved February 7, 2010 from http://www.sptimes.com/2005/08/21/Tampa bay/Making_a_difference_0.shtml

Todi, S. (2010). Sepsis:New Horizons. Indian Journal of Critical Care Medicine, 14, 1-2. Retrieved January 28, 2010 from http:/www.ijcm.org/text.asp?2010/14/1/63026

Todi, S., Chatterjee, S., Bhattacharyya, M. (2007). Epidemiology of severe sepsis in India. Critical Care 11, (Suppl2) : P65. Retrieved January 28, 2010 from http://www.ccforum/content/II/S2/P65

Todi, S., Chatterjee, S., Sahu, S., & Bhattacharyya (2010). Epidemiology of severe sepsis in India: an up-date. Critical Care, 14, (Suppl1) : P382. Retrieved January 28, 2010, from http://www.ncbi.nlm.nih.gov/pmc/articles/ PMC2934428

Toussaint, S., & Gerlach, H. (2009). Activated Protein C for Sepsis. New England Journal of Medicine, 361,2646-2652.

University of Brighton. (2010). Filtering Out Sepsis. Retrieved March 19, 2010 from http://www.brighton. acuk/research/health/casesstudy3.php?Pageld=274

Videojug Corporation. (2010). Epidemiology Basics: What is the basic premise of epidemiology? Retrieved January 23, 2010 from http://www.videojug.com/expertanswer/ epidemiology-basics-2/what-is-the-basic-premise-of-epidemiology

Wheat, H.W. (2010). Medicine in Virginia During the Civil War. Retrieved February 9, 2010 from http://www. encyclopediavirginia.org/Medicine_in_Virginia_During_ the_Civil_War.

Whiteman, H. & deMoura, H. (2009). Brazilian amputee model dead at 20. Retrieved February 6, 2010 from http://www.edition.cnn.com/2009?WORLD/americas/01 /24/brazil.amputee.model/index.html?iref=hpmostpop

Wikipedia Encyclopedia (n.d.). Dream: Dreams and psychosis. Retrieved February 22, 2010 from http://en.wikipedia.org/wiki/Dream

Wikipedia Encyclopedia. (n.d.). Epidemiology. Retrieved January 22, 2010 from http://www.en.wikipedia.org/ wiki/Epidemiology

Wikipedia Encyclopedia. (n.d.) Jim Henson. Retrieved February 5, 2010 from http://www.enwikipedia.org/ wiki/Jim_Henson

Winters, B.D., Eberlein, M.,Leung, J., Needham, D.M., Pronovost, P.J., & Sevransky, J.E. (2010). Long-term mortality and quality of life in sepsis: a systematic review. Critical Care Medicine, 38, 1276-1283. doi : 10.1097/CCM.0b013e3181d8cc1d

Yen, S., & Angus, D.C. (2007). Long-term Outcomes from Sepsis. Current Infectious Disease Reports, 9, 382-386.

**<u>Special thanks to the kind and generous
contributors that helped to make this book possible.</u>**

Jennifer Alford
Arlene Alleyne
Scott Andrews
Donald & Sandra (Rudd) Barnes
Adrian & Dorian & Gary & Nancy Black
Randall Brown
Yvonne Carswell
Thomas "Dale" Churchill
Robin Clapp
Tim Clarke & Linda Grandstaff
Jennifer Claro
Sherry Compton
Steve Daniel
Nicholas Darone
Carl L. & Hannah L.Darrisaw
Fred & Brenda Davis
Bill Davis
Lou Deroscher
Russell Diggs
Lisa Dove
Jimmy Duckett
Monique Feliciano
Jeff Flannery
Steve Gifford & Marie
Mr. Dennis Graves
Mrs. Felicia Graves
John Gregory IV
Tony Grimes

George F. Jr. &Antoinette W. Hamner
Bob & Eula (Bass) Helping
Roy C. & Jane B. Howard
Don & Kate Jones
Jeremy Jones
Kim Jones
Michael Keith
Kathleen & Kelvin Knipl
Ron & Jackie Koepke
William Larkin
Derek Lowery
Joan Mares
Kim Martin
Chuck & Evelyn Masuicca
Danielle McClean
Larry McEachern
Richard Mercereau
Joseph Micchia, MD
Cheque Miles
Amanda Miller
Bo & Lynn & Kari Miller
Cedric Miller
Sumuna Nekindinga
Howard G. Norris
Andy Offutt
Margaret Patton
Lawrence Perry
Kenny Plimphn
Shirley A Purvis

Nathan & Bonnie Richards
Jeremy & Shela Richards
Michael & Cindy & Melani Richards
Rick & Chris Richards
Anthony Robinson
Dave Robinson
Scott Robinson
Frank & Janell Rock
Mike Rockwood
Thomas Rooney (TOS)
Kyle Seitz
Irina Shiyanovskaya & Sergiy V. & Yuriy Shiyanovskii
Chimease Smith
Stranger (lady) at IGA
Adrian Sutton
Rose Marie Thomas
David Tuttle
Richard T. & Jo Anne L. Vacca
Sue Walker
Vegas Warren
Julius West
Harold E. Wilcox, PH D
Greg Wootton